MULTIPLE SCLEROSIS
A Guide for Patients and Their Families

MULTIPLE SCLEROSIS
A Guide for Patients and Their Families

Editor

Labe C. Scheinberg, M.D.

Professor of Neurology and Rehabilitation Medicine
Albert Einstein College of Medicine
Yeshiva University
Bronx, New York

Raven Press ■ New York

Raven Press, 1140 Avenue of the Americas, New York, New York 10036

Made in the United States of America

Library of Congress Cataloging in Publication Data
Main entry under title:

Multiple sclerosis.

   Bibliography: p. 241
   Includes indexes.
   1. Multiple sclerosis.   I. Scheinberg, Labe C.
[DNLM: 1. Multiple sclerosis—Popular works.   WL 360
M9563]
RC377.M843   1983   616.8′34   83-10995
ISBN 0-89004-776-6
ISBN 0-89004-960-2 *(paperback)*

The material contained in this volume was submitted as previously unpublished material, except in the instances in which credit has been given to the source from which some of the illustrative material was derived.

Great care has been taken to maintain the accuracy of the information contained in the volume. However, Raven Press cannot be held responsible for errors or for any consequences arising from the use of the information contained herein.

*This book is dedicated to our patients and to the late
Dr. Arthur S. Abramson, who taught us about
Multiple Sclerosis*

Foreword

Multiple sclerosis is the most common cause of neurological disability that attacks women and men in their productive years, between the ages of 15 and 55. About 90% have their onset in this age range. It is rare to contract multiple sclerosis before age 15 or after 55.

It is frequently a disease of tragic consequences—tragic both in the common meaning of that word and in the Aristotelian sense, providing as it often does "the spectacle of a virtuous man brought from prosperity to adversity," and inciting both terror and pity.

Multiple sclerosis is, after trauma and arthritic disorders, the most important cause of severe disability of adult life. Because of the long life expectancy of its victims, there are few, if any, conditions that have a greater socioeconomic impact.

It attacks individuals either during the late stages of education and training or just as they have embarked on establishing a family and/or career. Generally it strikes persons who are healthy, intelligent, and well educated—those to whom the future seems exceptionally bright. It cannot be attributed to any known "failing" or cause; and, again like the Greek tragedy, it too often imposes terrible penalties.

Multiple sclerosis is a chronic illness that affects most motor and sensory functions of the nervous system. Pain and loss of mental faculties are rare. It varies in severity and allows some to lead full, productive lives, whereas others are rendered totally helpless within a few years.

The cause of multiple sclerosis is unknown, but it is now thought to be the result of an abnormal response of the body to persistent infections. Much of the current research is directed along these lines. Moreover, there is no specific treatment, and nothing alters its unpredictable course. Attacks and remissions come without warning, confusing both patients and their families and making them prey to the many fad treatments that are, sadly, always available in such circumstances.

Only through research into the cause and mechanism of symptom development can we hope to find a prevention or cure for this disease. This difficult and costly approach often seems inefficient, but so long as one individual is crippled the search for a cure must continue. Sometimes answers come unexpectedly from seemingly unrelated fields within basic biomedical research; more often this route is slow and arduous.

In the meantime, health care teams continue to offer symptomatic treatment to the multiple sclerosis person to prevent or alleviate painful, disabling, and potentially life-shortening complications, as well as counseling and support to the person affected and his or her family. Moreover, there are enough resources in our society to carry on a forceful research program and to provide medically appropriate symptomatic treatment, particularly if these are not wasted on un-proved therapies and quackery.

This book is intended as a guide to patients and their families. It is a comprehensive, multidisciplinary approach, and those who have contributed to it have had long experience in dealing with the prob-lems described herein.

Multiple sclerosis with its varied complications is frustrating to the patient, the family, and the health practitioner. However, through the consistent and cooperative effort of all three, in collaboration with the National Multiple Sclerosis Society and other interested agencies, the answers will come. Until that time, we must be in-creasingly concerned with better management of the day-to-day problems encountered by the person who has multiple sclerosis.

S. Lawry

Acknowledgments

The contributors wish to acknowledge the editorial assistance of Jeanne Fogg.

Royalties from the sale of this book are being contributed to the Education Committee of the National Multiple Sclerosis Society.

Contents

Contributors

Arthur S. Abramson, M.D.
(Deceased)
Department of Rehabilitation Medicine
Albert Einstein College of Medicine
1300 Morris Park Avenue
Bronx, New York 10461

Justin Alexander, Ph.D.
Department of Rehabilitation Medicine
Albert Einstein College of Medicine
1300 Morris Park Avenue
Bronx, New York 10461

Diann Geronemus, M.S.W.,
ACSW
Consultant
National Multiple Sclerosis Society
2700 S.W. 4th Avenue
Fort Lauderdale, Florida 33315

Barbara S. Giesser, M.D.
Department of Neurology
Albert Einstein College of Medicine
1300 Morris Park Avenue
Bronx, New York 10461

Nancy J. Holland, M.A., R.N.
Multiple Sclerosis Comprehensive
 Care Center
Albert Einstein College of Medicine
1300 Morris Park Avenue
Bronx, New York 10461

Rosalind Kalb, Ph.D.
Departments of Neurology and
 Rehabilitation Medicine
Albert Einstein College of Medicine
1300 Morris Park Avenue
Bronx, New York 10461

Seymour R. Kaplan, M.D.
Department of Psychiatry
Albert Einstein College of Medicine
1300 Morris Park Avenue
Bronx, New York 10461

Nicholas G. LaRocca, Ph.D.
Department of Neurology
 (Psychology)
Albert Einstein College of Medicine
1300 Morris Park Avenue
Bronx, New York 10461

Sylvia Lawry
National Multiple Sclerosis Society
205 E. 42nd Street
New York, New York 10017

Margaret McDonnell, M.A.,
R.N.
Nursing Services
Good Samaritan Hospital
Pottsville, Pennsylvania 17901

Charles M. Poser, M.D.
Department of Neurology
Boston University Medical Center
80 E. Concord Street
Boston, Massachusetts 02118

Kay Robbins, M.A., OTR
Multiple Sclerosis Comprehensive
 Care Center
Albert Einstein College of Medicine
1300 Morris Park Avenue
Bronx, New York 10461

Labe Scheinberg, M.D.
Department of Neurology and
 Rehabilitation Medicine
Albert Einstein College of Medicine
1300 Morris Park Avenue
Bronx, New York 10461

James Simmons, M.D.
Consultant
67 Monterey Circle
Lavalette, New Jersey 08735
 and
National Multiple Sclerosis Society
205 E. 42nd Street
New York, New York 10017

Robert J. Slater, M.D.
National Multiple Sclerosis Society
205 E. 42nd Street
New York, New York 10017

Lola Sprinzeles, Ph.D., C.R.C.
Formerly at:
Department of Psychiatry
Albert Einstein College of Medicine
Bronx, New York 10461

Currently at:
588 West End Avenue
New York, New York 10024

John Whitaker, M.D.
1030 Jefferson Avenue
Memphis, Tennessee 38104
 and
Department of Neurology
University of Tennessee
Memphis, Tennessee 38104

Phyllis Wiesel-Levison,
 B.S., R.N.
Multiple Sclerosis Comprehensive
 Care Center
Albert Einstein College of Medicine
1300 Morris Park Avenue
Bronx, New York 10461

Leon Zitzer
Attorney General's Office
2 World Trade Center, 46th Floor
New York, New York 10047

People who want to make a living from the treatment of nervous patients must clearly be able to do something to help them.

Sigmund Freud

Many attempts have been made to find a causal and preventive treatment for multiple sclerosis, but they all have failed and are, therefore, rather illustrative of empirical trials based on more or less vaguely founded working hypotheses. This fact often led to one of two opposite prejudicial attitudes, which were more common earlier, but still are sadly prevalent. One of these represents the nihilistic attitude towards any kind of measure for helping the patients: "I am sorry, but there is no treatment, so I cannot help you." And the other one is the optimistic and magical belief in having found out the key method for curing the disease: "Come to me, I have elaborated a new method to treat multiple sclerosis and I have already cured hundreds of patients." There is today only one attitude to the multiple sclerosis patients, worthy of a neurologist and that is: "I cannot cure your disease but it may run a benign course and anyhow I will try to help you, because much can be done to make life easier for you."

Tore Broman
Department of Neurology
University of Gothenburg

MULTIPLE SCLEROSIS
A Guide for Patients and Their Families

1

Introduction

Labe Scheinberg

The organization of this book is traditional, beginning with a section on the possible causes (etiologies) and development (pathogenesis) of multiple sclerosis (MS). Current hypotheses concerning the origin of MS are presented along with possible contributing factors. The remaining sections are more clinical with a discussion of diagnosis and management by medical, surgical, physical, and psychological methods. The patients' problems are foremost, whether these are questions of diet, employment, sex, physical therapy, social adaptation, or unproved therapies.

If one were to ask for a brief description of MS, one could probably best reply, "It is an unpredictable neurologic disorder (disease of the nervous system) with its onset in early adult life, mostly affecting walking and often with associated urinary problems." There are of course visual and other sensory symptoms, fatigue, psychological problems, sexual difficulties, etc., but the major disability is in the area of mobility. All of these problems are discussed in detail.

MS is common enough to have earned the title of "the great crippler of young adults." Although the exact number of cases in the United States is unknown, it must approximate 200,000. After arthritis and trauma, it is the chief cause of major disability in adults of working age, that is, those between 16 and 60. The overall economic, social, and psychosexual implications are overwhelming in many instances. Because MS strikes individuals in their most productive years, just when they are assuming major family and career responsibilities, its impact may be greater than that of any other physical illness.

The cause of MS is unknown, and there is no specific treatment to cure MS, halt its progress, prevent attacks, or reverse longstanding damage. Although it is not possible to predict the course or outcome in an individual case, the outlook is better than generally believed. The average life expectancy is over 35 years after onset and has increased 10 to 15 years during the last few decades as the result of better medical care, especially of complications. The majority of MS persons are ambulatory, and many are gainfully employed even after 20 years.

There are several poorly understood features of MS: It seems to have a predilection for females (2:1 or 3:1). It also has a predilection for northern or moderate climates (it is about three times more prevalent in the temperate zones of Europe and North American than in the subtropical zones); it is very uncommon in the tropical and subtropical zones of the northern and southern hemispheres. It is rare in Asian and African countries. These features are provocative but poorly understood, with much epidemiological research under way to explain these geographic and racial or ethnic differences. There seems to be a greater prevalence in countries where the level of sanitation is higher. These unexplained differences are interesting and offer potential clues as to course and prevention, but they do not contribute to the care of the patient with MS.

MS necessitates intervention by many health professionals: neurologists, internists, primary care physicians, physiatrists, urologists, ophthalmologists, psychiatrists, surgeons, nurses, social workers, psychologists, physical therapists, occupational therapists, and others. Legal assistance is sometimes necessary to obtain disability benefits, remove architectural barriers, and prevent or correct discrimination in employment. The care of some patients may be overwhelming and frustrating to the family, and at times it may tax the resources of the solitary practitioner. Often a coordinated team is necessary to deliver continuing comprehensive care.

There are many ways to classify MS. It may be divided on the basis of certainty of diagnosis: that it is clinically definite, probable, or possible (suspected). It may be classified on the basis of course: benign, progressive, chronic relapsing, exacerbating and remitting, or plateau (stable). The location in the nervous system of the majority of lesions leading to the most significant disability has also been the basis of classification. These classifications all have their uses and are discussed more later.

Another important way of describing and understanding MS is to consider the psychosocial phases of the illness. Each phase may be characterized by the interactions of patient, family, and physician. The *first phase* is one of "uncertainty" and extends from the onset of the initial symptoms to the time of diagnosis. This is often difficult to measure because of its variable and often insidious onset as well as the lack of any specific diagnostic test. Some doctors believe that the disease cannot be diagnosed in most instances. Today the diagnosis is easier to make because of advances in radiology, evoked response testing (a clinical test measuring time of response of the brain to visual, auditory, or touch stimulation), and laboratory tests on the cerebrospinal fluid.

The *second phase* is one of "shock and settling in" and involves the physician informing the patient and family of the diagnosis. Some physicians are reluctant to inform the patient, and when they do such terms as "chronic viral infection of the nervous system," "allergic reaction," "demyelinating disease," etc. are used. The reasons for this reluctance vary from an uncertainty of the diagnosis, an unwillingness to tell a patient the diagnosis when no treatment is available, or the fear that the patient may be made worse by the emotional shock of learning the diagnosis. I believe that the patient should be informed of the diagnosis when it is established and the term "multiple sclerosis" and "MS" be employed. Only in this way will the patient be able to establish a relationship of trust with the physician, obtain the assistance available, and plan the future in a meaningful way.

Failure to inform the patient may result in additional and unnecessary consultations, more diagnostic tests, and especially anxiety. Many patients, when questioned later, express relief at having finally learned the diagnosis because they had suspected a more malignant disease or a psychiatric disorder. Associated with learning the diagnosis is the "settling-in" period, which may be characterized by denial, anxiety, hostility, depression, bewilderment, or even relief. These reactions can be ameliorated by a thorough, frank discussion of MS and education of the patient and family about all aspects of MS. The patient must be supported during this period by a concerned, candid physician.

The *third phase* is "early treatment," often with adrenocortical steroids (cortisone and similar drugs) or pituitary hormone (ACTH), which may shorten an attack, although the evidence that this is so is not convincing. Remissions occur frequently within weeks, even without treatment, and may be complete.

The *fourth phase*, or *chronic care phase*, usually begins a few months after diagnosis and may last for decades. During this period the patient may lose confidence in the initial practitioner and seek medical care from others or resort to "fad therapy." Financial and emotional costs can be staggering. The patient may become unemployed, and family breakdowns or other psychosocial tragedies may occur. Chronic care in a hospital is the final course in some severe cases.

During this phase resources must be gathered to support the patient and family. With no specific treatment available, the best that can be done is to manage the symptoms and minimize complications, such as urinary tract infections or contractures. We have learned that the most valuable adjunct to care is a stable personality and supportive family or friends. Because one cannot easily alter personality and because supportive relationships may be absent, the only alternative is to try to provide substitute resources.

This book is intended as a general guide for those who suffer with MS and those who care for them. It is intended to be a guide on ways to adapt to an unpredictable illness and to lead a long and productive life in spite of it. There are few references or footnotes, but a general reading list is provided. Some sections use terminology that is familiar, and reading will be easy. Others may require some study, however. We make the assumption that the average patient with MS is intelligent, curious, and concerned. The book is slanted toward that reader. The aim is to answer some questions and, hopefully, help those who live with MS to lead healthier, more productive lives.

2

What Causes the Disease?

John N. Whitaker

Multiple sclerosis (MS) is a disease in which the insulation surrounding nerve fibers of the central nervous system (the brain and
spinal cord) is damaged. Tissue outside the central nervous system
is not involved in the disease. Infections of the urinary and respi-
ratory systems, which are commonly seen in persons with MS, are
simply complications of MS.

Although knowledge about the factors influencing the development of MS has increased appreciably during the last decade, its
cause is basically unknown. We can speculate, however, and offer
here some possible causes. In addition, the basic damage that occurs
within the body must be understood so that the MS individual and
his or her family can better cope with the disorder.

WHY THE SYMPTOMS?

In order to identify the pathological changes which explain the
symptoms in patients with MS, it is necessary to understand some
of the anatomy of the central nervous system (CNS). This system
is characterized by the specialized activities of its component cells.
Actions and reactions of the individual's body depend on "news"
of the stimulus being transmitted to the brain, the brain's reaction,
and "instructions" on how to react to the stimulus then being sent
from the brain back to the original point. This coordinated transmission of a nerve impulse from one nerve cell to the next underlies
nervous tissue function and is dependent on the connections among
the nerve cells. These "connections" are called nerve fibers. The
coordination among these nerve cells is a result of the integrity and
the speed of conduction of an impulse along the nerve fiber to the

synapse (connection point) to the next nerve cell. Myelin (a fatty substance that surrounds the nerve fiber, forming a sheath) enhances the velocity with which nerve impulses are conducted along the fibers.

The conduction of an impulse along an axon may be viewed as similar to the movement of current in an electrical wire. Myelin provides the insulation around nerve fibers and allows only a small portion of the nerve fiber membrane to become depolarized (change in electrical charge) and the impulse to be transmitted. The presence of the myelin sheath markedly reduces any leakage of "current."

In MS this sheath is damaged so that the insulation can no longer prevent leakage. As a result, transmission may either cease completely or be delayed. In either event, a nervous system activity (such as vision, strength, sensation, or coordination) is lost or diminished because of the block or delay in impulse transmission.

The initial lesion (area of abnormality) in MS that leads to the tissue alterations (myelin damage) is still unclear. However, it is known that the myelin breaks down in the presence of certain cells, and in the absence of myelin certain other cells proliferate and form dense tissue at the site of the damage. This proliferation causes a firmness of the tissue (sclerosis). Sclerotic tissue is similar to scar tissue. The loss of myelin, the sclerosis, and the fact that the lesions occur in many sites throughout the CNS account for the name "multiple," or "disseminated," sclerosis.

There are areas of inflammation in MS which are usually characterized by the accumulation of cells, especially in the early phases of the disease; these cells usually accumulate around blood vessels in the CNS. It is not known how or why they arrive at the site where they eventually gather and form a lesion. It *is* known, however, that they both injure the tissue and digest (phagocytize) the damaged myelin.

Another cell which appears to be related to this inflammatory collection but which remains within the CNS for a long period of time is the "plasma cell." This cell produces immunoglobulin, which is a protein in the serum that contains antibodies. The "plasma cells" found within brain tissue of persons with MS may produce large amounts of gamma globulin (also called immunoglobulin). As this material may then spill into the cerebrospinal fluid and its presence can be detected by laboratory tests, its presence is used to help in the diagnosis of MS.

The damage to myelin in nerve cells, which is seen when tissues are examined after death, is usually more extensive than was suggested by the symptoms seen during life. Hence it appears that there are attacks in patients that have not produced symptoms severe enough to be felt by the patient or seen by the doctor. That these subclinical attacks occur means that there is no clear way to predict the course of tissue injury in this disease, as the extent of the damage can be seen only after death.

WHAT CAUSES THE DAMAGE?

The basic features of MS were described over 100 years ago. Those observations and the ones made subsequently which have bearing on the cause of MS may be summarized as follows: MS is an acquired, inflammatory, primary breakdown of certain tissues in the CNS that occurs in multiple and random sites. Cellular overgrowth and a fibrotic response within these areas account for the sclerosis. It is uncertain how the disease then progresses, although we know that there is often subclinical involvement which goes undetected until an autopsy is performed. No absolutely specific diagnostic tests are yet available. However, there are now methods that measure certain components in the cerebrospinal fluid which indicate recent tissue damage and immunological studies that provide an indication about the mechanism. Both environmental influences and host (the person with the disease) factors, especially those involving the immune system, apparently contribute to the development of MS.

When seeking the cause of MS and the mechanisms by which it develops, it is helpful to focus on three areas: the influences of the environment, the immune system, and the characteristics of certain tissues of the CNS.

The Environment

Geographic Factors

One of the most puzzling facts about MS is its uneven geographic distribution. There is a wide prevalence of MS (30 to 80 cases per 100,000 population) in the northern, temperate zones in North America and Europe as well as in the southern portions of New Zealand and Australia. The disease occurs less frequently in countries near the equator. The most striking exception to this distribution is in Japan. Although some of Japan's islands lie at latitudes that should be in zones of high prevalence, MS rarely appears there: There are only about two cases of MS per 100,000 population in Japan.

The particular geographic distribution of MS may indicate an environmental influence, but it could also be the result of genetic factors of the European peoples who subsequently populated the high-prevalence zones. Certain racial groups, notably Orientals and to a lesser extent blacks, within these temperate latitudes have a low or lower incidence of MS than whites within the same regions.

Geographic differences in the prevalence of MS have afforded the opportunity of examining variables within the environment. For example, the Shetland, Orkney, and Faeroe Islands lie to the north of Scotland within several degrees of latitude of each other, but the prevalence of MS among people living on the Orkneys and the Shetlands is more than twice that found on the Faeroes. These differences have been variably interpreted to be due to the presence of an infectious agent, dietary differences, or contaminated water supplies. However, there is no proof that any of these factors are responsible.

There has been no major change in prevalence of the disease in the United States over the past few decades. In some countries it is impossible to determine if the incidence of MS is the same or has changed. This is because of the mobility of the population or the incompletely kept health records. In other areas, however, there are enough figures available to say that MS epidemics are in force.

One of these areas is the Faeroe Islands. Here no new cases of MS were reported from 1920 to 1943, but between 1943 and 1977 there were 25 new cases, with 24 of them beginning during the interval 1943 to 1960. The explanation for this outbreak may be related to the fact that British troops occupied the Faeroe Islands during 1940 to 1945 as part of their wartime duties. Thus, although possibly coincidental, it appears that the disease-inducing agents accounting for the sudden appearance of the MS may have been brought by the British soldiers.

Age

MS typically begins in persons 15 to 50 years of age, but there are indications from individuals who move from one area to another that an environmental influence is exerted during childhood. Studies have shown that in immigrants to South Africa and Israel, for example, where they lived prior to age 15 affects their chances of having MS many years later.

Conclusions

These environmental relationships suggest that viruses, toxins, or nutritional deficiency may be factors in the disease. However, although a number of toxins (poisons) and certain vitamin-deficiency states may lead to nerve damage, the abnormal alterations in the CNS caused by these agents are different from those seen in MS; moreover, in these conditions there are often changes in the peripheral nervous system that do not occur in MS.

There is no direct evidence that an environmental pollutant causes MS or that vitamins are in any way active in the prevention or arrest of MS. In terms of the environment, then, the strongest candidate is an infectious agent.

Genetic Predisposition

An individual's genetic inheritance may influence whether he or she ultimately develops MS. This statement is based on the fact that there is a 12- to 20-fold increase in the frequency of MS among first-degree relatives (those in the immediate family) of the MS victim. It is important to remember, though, that the genetic effect manifests itself as one which increases the *predisposition* for acquiring the disease rather than dictating a definite pattern of inheritance. Thus *the disease itself is not actually transmitted genetically.*

Human cells normally contain 46 chromosomes, on which reside genes that control the production of all body components. Markers for a predisposition to MS have been sought by analyzing genetically determined tissue components. Except for identical twins, antigens differ among individuals. (Antigens are substances which stimulate antibody production. Antibodies are substances in the immune system which "attack" alien substances, or antigens, in the body.) On exposure to a foreign, or non-self, antigen, the person's immune system recognizes the antigen and mounts a response to reject it (called an immune response).

Since the advent of organ transplantation and the need to match donors and recipients for compatibility, identification of the genes controlling tissue-compatible antigens has progressed at a rapid pace. It has been demonstrated in some population groups, notably those of Northern European ancestry, that there is a two- to fourfold increase in the frequency of certain antigens (designated HLA-A3, HLA-B7, and HLA-Dw2) in patients with MS compared to normal persons. However, there is no rigid association between the known HLA types and the presence of MS. For example, persons with MS may have none of the HLA types that have been shown to occur frequently in persons with MS. Conversely, the "predisposing" HLA types may be present without MS. As a corollary to this, laboratory procedures utilizing these facts cannot yet be used to predict who might or might not develop MS.

At what point in MS genetic factors are involved is unknown, but this is obviously an important question. The chromosome sites that determine which HLA types are present lie near the genes that control the immune response (see the next section). Hence a genetic influence could be related to some immune response to an infectious agent or to the body's autoimmune response to some substance within itself that the body (for some unknown reason) suddenly decides is not acceptable.

The Immune System

An "immune response" in any individual, with or without a specific disease, simply refers to the body reacting to a foreign agent (virus, bacteria, etc.) to protect itself against that agent. Occasionally the body goes "haywire" and starts to react against its own tissues. This is called an "autoimmune response."

The host's immune system may be involved in the onset or perpetuation of MS. Cells of lymphoid tissue (thymus, spleen, lymph nodes, certain blood cells) generate and control an immune response. In man most of the information has been obtained from studies of lymphocytes (certain blood cells), which are readily accessible for analysis. These lymphocytes have several specialized functions. Some produce and secrete antibody or directly attack and destroy an infectious organism; these are "effector" cells. Others help promote an immune response or suppress it; these are "regulatory" cells.

Investigation of the general immune status of persons with MS has disclosed no consistent abnormality in the blood, although when more specific and sensitive tests are used regulatory lymphocytes have been found to be abnormal. That is, there is a decrease or disappearance of these lymphocytes from the peripheral blood at the very time MS exacerbates. The number of these cells returns to normal or above normal when the patient goes into remission. Whether these cells are destroyed, enter the CNS, or merely alter their circulatory route in the body remains to be determined. It is also unclear how an alteration of this type would manifest as MS, but the correlation of the cyclic changes in clinical symptoms and the number of these cells in the bloodstream is intriguing.

Cerebrospinal Fluid

It has been known for more than 35 years that there is usually an increase in the amount of gamma globulin in the cerebrospinal fluid of persons with MS. (Gamma globulin is now called immunoglobulin, a more specific scientific designation, and IgG is the predominant immunoglobulin.)

Cerebrospinal fluid normally contains up to 45 milligrams of protein per 100 milliliters. IgG constitutes less than 15% of the total amount of protein present. As noted, in persons with MS the IgG in the cerebrospinal fluid is increased, which results primarily because of the production of IgG by certain cells ("plasma cells") within the CNS. These cells appear to arise from blood lymphocytes, which enter the CNS when the MS patient is having bouts of inflammatory nerve damage. When examined by suitable techniques, the cerebrospinal fluid proteins of the vast majority (80 to 90%) of persons with MS show selective increases of certain forms of IgG, but the presence of these forms of IgG in cerebrospinal fluid is not specific for MS; they are found in other diseases as well. In association with the changes in IgG in the cerebrospinal fluid, antibodies to a number of viruses are also found to be increased. However, neither of these conditions is specific for MS or even precisely parallels the disease's activity.

Viruses and MS

Viruses or other infectious agents have been suspected for many years to be the cause of MS. As different infectious organisms have been discovered and identified, they have been examined for a possible linkage to MS. During the past 20 years attention to an infectious basis for MS has been directed primarily at viruses.

Numerous types of virus exist with an array of features that determine how they infect and alter tissue. The behavior of the virus is the result of a virus's own characteristics and the cells to which it is exposed. A host cell may show a number of reactions in response to a viral infection, ranging from minimal or no change to malignant transformation to death. In addition to the changes produced by the usual type of virus, mutant viruses may appear which have different characteristics of infectivity or disease induction.

Evidence for viral involvement in MS or any condition can be sought using several methods. The most convincing is the culture, isolation, and identification of a virus in tissues taken from areas of damage. Other methods include recognizing parts of a virus in tissue and detecting antibodies (which would attack that particular virus) in the blood or cerebrospinal fluid of those affected. Finding the antibody would indicate that the person had been exposed to the virus at one time or another.

The virus that causes measles (rubeola) has been analyzed extensively as the possible cause of MS. This measles virus is known also to cause a chronic nervous system disease of childhood called subacute sclerosing panencephalitis. Beginning in 1962 it was recognized that persons with MS have increased amounts of antibody to the measles virus in their bloodstream. Although a number of studies have confirmed this observation and have also shown that some of the antibody to measles is being produced by the CNS, evidence for the measles virus also causing MS remains highly circumstantial.

Dogs and MS

Even less convincing than the information on measles is the relationship between exposure to dogs and the development of MS. This is an emotional and highly controversial issue on which opinions differ greatly. Canine distemper is a viral infection that produces an inflammatory disease of the CNS in dogs, and the canine distemper virus has a number of characteristics in common with the measles virus. Even though the case for incriminating dogs and/or canine distemper in the development of MS is not strong, an effective program for the vaccination of dogs against canine distemper should be followed.

Slow Virus

When attempting to relate environmental influences from 10 to 20 years before to the appearance of MS now, a "slow virus" must be considered. In contrast to the usual acute or subacute response to conventional viruses, "slow viruses" cause diseases that may evolve over a period of months to years. One of these viruses induces an inflammatory CNS disease in sheep, but there is no indication that any one of the known "slow viruses" causes MS.

Other Viruses

Several conventional viruses have been identified as causing a CNS disease in animals that shows some of the same tissue changes as are seen in MS. Hence because of the many mechanisms whereby a virus might inflict CNS damage, a viral etiology for MS has by no means been excluded.

3

The Diagnosis

Charles M. Poser

Although some laboratory tests have been developed, the diagnosis of MS is still based on clinical evidence. The physician must be able to show that there are two or more abnormalities (lesions) of the central nervous system (the brain and spinal cord), that these lesions predominantly involve the white matter of the brain, and that other illnesses that also produce multiple lesions have been ruled out. Depending largely on the severity and duration of the disease, these findings can vary from being extremely easy to extremely difficult to confirm.

Because the diagnosis remains essentially a clinical one—based on symptoms and signs of the individual's nervous system malfunction, it is highly dependent on how accurate the individual's medical history is and the physician's skill in eliciting and properly evaluating this information.

A *symptom* is something that is noted by the patient. This may be a change in sensation or loss of it, weakness of a body part, a lessening of vision, pain, or clumsiness. A *sign* is an abnormality detected by the physician while examining the person. At times signs confirm the presence of symptoms. For example, a physician may be able to detect the weakness or delineate the sensory loss of which the patient complains. On the other hand, abnormal nervous system signs such as nystagmus (an oscillating movement of the eyes), abnormal reflexes such as the Babinski sign (when the sole of the foot is scratched the toe extends) or loss of vibratory sense may be present without the patient being aware of anything being wrong. In essence, symptoms are subjective complaints, whereas signs are objective observations. The patient must search his or her memory and often turn to friends and close relatives in order to recall symptoms that may be significant. Finally, the physician must select certain procedures and laboratory tests that confirm that the patient does indeed have a medical abnormality that causes his or her symptoms. These various tests often also provide evidence of the existence of multiple abnormal areas (lesions) in the nervous system.

PROBLEMS OF CLINICAL DIAGNOSIS

There are many difficulties inherent in the recall of symptoms by the individual and their interpretation by the doctor before a diagnosis of MS can be established. Symptoms may be decidedly transient, lasting not just hours or days but sometimes only minutes. They are often bizarre and so may be dismissed as irrelevant or not significant by both patient and physician. Because symptoms may be mild and fleeting they are often easily forgotten.

Although information on the symptoms of MS is easily available to the public in specially prepared materials, many physicians have little experience with this disease and so misinterpret the symptoms and make incorrect diagnoses. Medical terminology is also often confusing both for the person affected and the physician. Other diseases that are called by the term "sclerosis" are sometimes confused with MS; for example, many people think that MS is the same as amyotrophic lateral sclerosis (Lou Gehrig's disease), although the two diseases have nothing in common whatsoever. The most common symptoms of MS are well known: numbness and tingling of an arm or leg, double or blurred vision, clumsiness of fine movements or of walking, and frequency and urgency of urination.

Unfortunately, many of these symptoms arise for other reasons. Blurring or graying of vision occurs far more often as a result of eye disease than it does because of the optic nerve inflammation that is characteristic of MS. True double vision (which is common in MS) is simply a sign that there is an imbalance of the muscles that control eye movement. As this movement is finely coordinated, anything that affects this extremely delicate balance will cause double vision; because true double vision (diplopia) is produced by both eyes it immediately disappears on closing *either* eye. Double vision that persists when one eye is shut, on the other hand, indicates some kind of functional or psychological disturbance. Diseases other than MS, such as myasthenia gravis or diabetes, also often cause double vision. People also experience double vision when they first start using bifocal glasses.

Numbness and paresthesias (pins-and-needles or prickly sensations, the sensations of a limb being asleep) are other common symptoms of MS that not infrequently occur in perfectly normal people. Hyperventilation (heavy breathing) is frequently followed by such sensations. Several commonly used medications, especially antidepressant drugs and diuretics ("water pills") often produce such abnormal sensations as side effects. Interference with blood circulation, as well as involvement of the peripheral nerves by conditions such as diabetes, a poorly functioning thyroid gland, and others may result in similar complaints. Strokes may also result in numbness that affects an entire side of the body or just one limb. Strokes, however, are more likely to occur in older persons who are past the usual age when MS is first seen. Sensory changes resulting from MS tend to be asymmetrical and to occur quite suddenly.

Incoordination of gait (walking) may result from overindulgence in alcohol or it may be a side effect of some commonly used drugs: tranquilizers, antihistamines, sedatives such as phenobarbital, and anticonvulsant drugs such as Dilantin. Incoordination of the fine movements of the hands is seen less frequently but may be associated with trembling; the latter condition is simply part of what is called "familial essential tremor," a completely benign condition that begins in youth.

Another source of confusion for both patients and physicians relates to disturbances of urinary bladder function. Frequency, urgency, and incontinence (loss of control of the bladder and rarely of the bowel) may indicate that certain parts of the spinal cord are affected by MS, but these symptoms may also be caused by a urinary tract or bladder infection. Bladder infections are often associated with pain and burning on urination, and these symptoms as well as nocturia (having to get up in the middle of the night to urinate) in

MS patients are frequently blamed on a bladder infection by both patient and physician when in fact there is no infection present.

Conversely, some symptoms are blamed on MS when in truth they are not usually seen with that disease. These include pain, headaches, convulsive seizures, sudden temporary loss of strength, and ringing in the ears. Dizziness (vertigo) is remarkably rare as an early symptom, as are sudden serious mental disturbances.

Weakness of an arm or leg, with or without sensory symptoms (any alteration of sensation, such as numbness or tingling) or incoordination, is frequent in MS but may of course indicate some other disturbance as well. If there is pain with the weakness, it is extremely unlikely that MS is at fault. One form of weakness—the rapidly developing, even quite sudden, paralysis of both lower extremities, often associated with loss of sensation in the legs—represents a peculiar manifestation of MS called "transverse myelitis," in which a lesion transects, or "cuts," the spinal cord, disturbing its function. This is usually seen in association with bladder and bowel paralysis.

Certain symptoms are so unusual they may puzzle both the patient and the physician. A sudden sensation of an electric shock running down the patient's back when the head is flexed suddenly is called Lhermitte's sign. Occasionally the same sensation is experienced when bending forward at the waist. It is often erroneously believed that Lhermitte's sign is positive proof of MS, whereas it actually indicates any disturbance very high in the spinal cord. Patients with MS sometimes lose their color vision for a few minutes and are unable to interpret traffic lights correctly at one corner but by the time they reach the next set of lights they have recovered the ability to distinguish red from green. The dubious expression on the unprepared physician's face when told such a story can easily be imagined!

In general, the disease is most difficult to diagnose in its earliest stages. Often symptoms are considered hysterical (caused by being overly emotional) when they are in fact real. Just as frequently, however, symptoms experienced by some individuals are inconsequential but are interpreted as being symptoms of MS.

THE DIAGNOSTIC PROCESS

Three elements are important to the process of arriving at a diagnosis: (a) the history obtained from the patient; (b) the neurological examination (tests of the nervous system); and (c) a variety of specialized procedures which may include examinations of the cerebrospinal fluid (the fluid that courses through the spinal column), certain types of X-rays, and a number of electrical tests.

The problems regarding the history have already been noted. It should be mentioned, however, that another important characteristic of MS, in addition to the presence of multiple, scattered lesions of the nervous system, is that in about two-thirds of MS patients symptoms come and go. These fluctuations are called exacerbations (when the symptoms are present) and remissions (when they are not). These periods are difficult to define, particularly in terms of severity and duration. During remissions symptoms do not always disappear completely. Often careful examination reveals that a symptom (for example, loss of sensation or the presence of a prickly sensation) has not disappeared but, rather, has become less noticeable so that the patient notes a relative improvement. In other situations, the patient has learned to compensate for and ignore what was at first an annoying symptom.

Several schemes for diagnosing MS have been proposed, and the one most frequently used in the United States is based on the Schumacher criteria. In most of the schemes for diagnosing MS, the disease is classified as "possible," "probable," and "definite" based on the physician's ability to demonstrate the presence of more than one lesion in the patient's central nervous system. Until recently, this determination had to be based almost exclusively on information garnered from the history and physical examination. Today, however, with the development of some specialized procedures, particularly measurement of a variety of evoked responses (the recording of electrical activity produced by the brain when it is stimulated by light or sound patterns) and computer-assisted tomography (CAT scanning, a special kind of X-ray), the diagnosis is more easily attained and is certainly more accurate. Nevertheless, in many instances the term "definite MS" must be viewed with care. There is as yet no absolutely reliable single laboratory procedure that can be performed on the patient, his blood, or his cerebrospinal fluid that by itself establishes the diagnosis of MS. Some laboratory tests almost do so but only when combined with information obtained from the history and physical examination.

Many diseases of the central nervous system, at their onset, have exactly the same symptoms and the same abnormalities on the physical examination, but these later prove to be significant for establishing the diagnosis of MS. Therefore it is often more valuable and certainly less expensive to simply observe the patient over a period of weeks or even months than to perform a series of diagnostic procedures that in the early stage of the disease may only indicate that *some* central nervous system disorder is present. For this reason, the category of "possible" MS is particularly difficult to define. It leaves the patient and quite often the physician in an uncomfortable state of indecision.

Once a diagnosis of MS has been made, it has to be confirmed. The diagnosis is generally established by obtaining evidence that different, widely separated areas of the central nervous system are affected. For example, a 25-year-old woman has double vision for 2 weeks, weakness of the left leg, numbness and a prickly sensation in her right arm for a month, and episodes of urinary frequency and urgency with several instances of loss of bladder control (incontinence)—all of these things appearing within a period of a few months. These signs and symptoms in themselves are sufficient to make the diagnosis. Simple confirmation may be obtained through a neurological examination, which shows that the patient has nystagmus (rapid oscillation of the eyeball), tendon reflexes that are more active on the right side than on the left, a lessened vibratory sense in the right hand, and a Babinski sign (testing of a reflex on the foot). Theoretically, the physician needs to look no further to be quite confident of the diagnosis. Usually, however, he or she will order one or more confirmatory tests. Today there are many tests that are noninvasive, completely harmless, and produce no discomfort whatsoever. It is no longer necessary to perform lengthy, painful, and expensive tests to confirm the diagnosis.

Neurological Examination

The neurological examination (of the nervous system) is the simplest and often the most convincing way of establishing or confirming the MS diagnosis. The disease affects certain parts of the central nervous system most often, causing characteristic symptoms and signs of abnormal functioning. The symptoms have already been mentioned. However, actual signs of dysfunction cannot always be related to symptoms, as many signs produce no alterations that can be felt or experienced by the patient.

It must also be emphasized that lesions that do not produce any symptom or even sign of malfunction exist in practically every MS patient. It is important for patients to realize this so that they understand that the appearance of a new symptom does not necessarily signify the formation of a new area of involvement. It is difficult to understand how lesions that are discovered at autopsy have not produced symptoms in view of their location and size, but they are seen repeatedly.

When the physician looks into the subject's eyes with his ophthalmoscope, he is examining that portion of the optic nerve that is visible as it penetrates the eyeball. In MS the optic nerve is often pale, suggesting that it may have been damaged earlier, but the damage did not cause any alteration of visual functions; alternatively, the damage may have produced such a transient visual disturbance that it has been forgotten by the patient. Nystagmus is often present. The patient may complain of double vision; the physician will then ask the individual to direct his eyes in various directions and note if both eyes do not move exactly together as they are supposed to do. Sometimes the physician can detect double vision of which the patient has not been aware.

Mild degrees of weakness and incoordination may be detected during the physical examination, as may slight changes in the subject's equilibrium when walking or standing. Examination of the sensory system is quite often disappointing. Despite the fact that the patient clearly describes a pins-and-needles sensation involving an arm or leg, a detailed examination of that limb may reveal no alteration of sensation. This is sometimes true even for such specialized senses as position (the relationship between the patient's body and space) or vibration (the ability to feel the vibration of a tuning apparatus placed on bony protrusions, such as the ankles or the fingers). Inequality in the activity of the reflexes on either side or determining that they are quite active is significant. The fact that the big toe goes up rather than down (the Babinski sign) when the outside of the sole of the foot is scratched with a sharp object indicates a disturbance of the major nervous pathways that carry messages from the brain to the muscles, even though the patient may not be aware of any symptom of such involvement.

The neurological (nervous system) examination is a way of further establishing the fact that a number of separate lesions exist within the central nervous system.

If the abdominal reflexes are absent (the abdominal muscles do not twitch when they are gently stroked with a sharp object), many neurologists consider this an important clue. Unfortunately, such reflexes tend to disappear normally in women who have had several pregnancies and in both men and women who are obese. Many neurological signs are caused by other conditions. Nystagmus, for example, often results from taking commonly prescribed medications, such as Valium, sleeping pills including most barbiturates, and many anticonvulsant drugs. Unequal reflexes (an abnormal finding) may result from injuries to the area where they are being tested, particularly the knees. The physician must be just as careful when interpreting the signs noted in the neurological examination as when he ascribes significance to symptoms and complaints related to him by the patient.

Simple Clinical Diagnostic Procedures

An important consideration in MS is the fact that some central nervous system lesions cause no symptoms. There are several techniques that can be used to detect these lesions. These tests are particularly important in patients whose clinical history and physical examination indicate that he has only a single lesion of the central nervous system. In such cases a search must be made for more lesions in order to confirm the diagnosis of MS.

A simple procedure which is quite useful either in the office or at the bedside is to look for unsuspected unilateral color blindness. Loss of the ability to distinguish colors, most frequently red and green, is very common in MS. It may be the only manifestation of optic neuritis (involvement of the optic nerve), which is a common feature of MS. Few patients are aware of this loss of color vision unless they accidentally shut one eye and discover that the other eye has become color-blind. The doctor can have the patient identify the "hidden" numbers in the Ishihara or AO pseudoisochromatic color plates in order to reveal such color blindness.

Another simple and extremely useful procedure is the hot-bath test, in which the patient is immersed in a bath at a temperature of 104°F (40°C) for 10 to 15 minutes. This test was devised because it has been demonstrated that the nerve fiber's ability to conduct an electrical impulse may become blocked when the temperature is elevated. In nerve fibers that have lost all or part of their insulatory myelin sheath (as happens in MS), the tolerance for temperature elevation is severely diminished; thus even very minor changes (as little as 0.1°C) will result in such blockage and symptoms will appear. This test not only can bring out symptoms that the patient has complained of in the past but does not feel at that moment, but it can also evoke symptoms that have never been noted before. In addition, signs of nervous system dysfunction may show up that are not present when the patient's temperature is normal. This test is particularly useful in persons who report that their symptoms are often aggravated or appear only when they are exposed to heat. For example, patients who sun themselves on the beach may notice that after 15 to 30 minutes they are unable to get up, develop double vision, or suddenly note pins-and-needles sensations in the right arm. These heat-induced symptoms disappear the moment the patient is cool. This observation is in fact the basis for the hot-bath test. When overheated, the patient may complain of symptoms of a lesion that has been present but "silent" for weeks, months, or years; he may notice a sudden decrease in visual acuity or double vision; he may be incoordinated when performing fine movements with his fingers; and he may be seen to have unilateral or bilateral Babinski signs that were not elicited previously. The hot-bath test is often sufficient to demonstrate the second lesion which is necessary to establish the diagnosis of MS.

Neurophysiological Tests

One of the greatest contributions to the diagnosis of MS has been the development of various techniques for recording and measuring evoked potentials. To explain: When light is flashed into the eyes, or a person is asked to look at a particular light stimulus (such as a black-and-white checkerboard on which the colors are reversed two times per second), electrical activity is produced in a specific part of the brain (the occipital lobe, where all visual impulses are recorded). This electrical activity can be recorded by the electroencephalograph (EEG), a machine that records brain waves. In order for this activity to be separated from the normal activity of the brain, the stimuli are repeated several hundred times; and the resulting brain activity (electrical impulses) is fed into a computer which manipulates the data so that they can be interpreted. The resultant activity is what is known as an evoked response, in this instance from visual stimuli. Similar information can be obtained by stimulating the ears with clicks (auditory evoked responses) or by stimulating nerves in the arm and in the legs (somatosensory evoked responses) and recording the resulting electrical impulses from the appropriate parts of the brain.

These procedures are extremely valuable, not only for confirming an already suspected lesion but, more importantly, for demonstrating a completely asymptomatic, unsuspected lesion. They have the advantage of being completely harmless to the patient. Measurement of both the visual and auditory evoked responses is painless, although measuring the somatosensory evoked responses may be uncomfortable because of the strength of the electrical current necessary to stimulate the nerves at the wrist or knee.

The visual evoked responses test is by far the most valuable; this is because it can demonstrate unsuspected lesions of the optic nerves in 75% of patients with MS who have never been aware of any previous alteration of vision. The other two procedures yield fewer positive results but still enough to warrant their use.

Another commonly used test is the Kimura blink reflex measurement. The test is carried out by measuring the time it takes for a mild stimulus to the eye to produce a blink of the eyelid. This test is also both painless and harmless, and is of diagnostic value in some patients with MS.

There are other more sophisticated but less frequently used tests involving vision. One of the more interesting and still not usually available tests measures contrast sensitivity. It helps to explain the blurring of vision that is seen in some patients with MS. Such blurring results from the eyes' loss of ability to differentiate between various contrasting shades. Another function that is often impaired in MS is the ability to fuse into a single stimulus flickers of light which are separated in time. This is called "impairment of flicker-fusion." Only very specialized laboratories are able to carry out these tests.

The EEG (brain wave test) itself, despite the unfortunate fact that it is frequently ordered in MS patients, is of no value whatsoever. When alterations are present, they are either totally irrelevant to the disease or are completely nonspecific and nondiagnostic. Similarly, electrical examination of nerve and muscle (electromyography) and nerve conduction testing is unwarranted unless either the history or the physical examination suggests involvement of the peripheral nervous system. (The central nervous system—the brain and spinal cord—can be viewed as the main control system of the body. The peripheral nervous system is composed of the nerves branching from the central system which carry messages to and from the central system. The peripheral nervous system is never involved in MS patients.) If there is a peripheral nervous system disturbance, such as a lesion of that system (perhaps as a result of trauma or an alcoholic or diabetic neuropathy), electromyography and/or nerve conduction time testing may be useful.

X-ray Examinations

X-ray examinations of the skull are of no value whatsoever, and brain scans are generally of little help. Computer-assisted tomography (CAT scanning, a special x-ray examination) is more valuable in determining the activity of the illness than in establishing the diagnosis. The procedure is very expensive and has a relatively low yield compared to the more productive evoked-response studies (see above). The CAT scan, however, may be able to demonstrate the presence of multiple lesions, necessary evidence on which to base the definitive diagnosis of MS. The new technique of nuclear magnetic resonance (NMR) is said to be more sensitive and safer than present procedures in diagnosis and will be widely available in a few years.

Myelography

Myelography is a procedure in which a heavy, oily material containing iodine is injected into the spinal canal in order to outline the spinal cord so it can be seen on an x-ray film. It has been said, only half jocularly, that many physicians feel safe in making the diagnosis of MS only after obtaining a negative myelogram. At best this test is unpleasant, but it also may have serious side effects. It is true that a high cervical (spinal cord) lesion (such as a tumor) may produce symptoms for a time which are like those of MS, including nystagmus. Usually, however, a careful review of the patient's history for visual problems and the demonstration of an abnormality of the visual evoked response abolish the need for a myelogram. The auditory evoked response, the Kimura blink reflex, and the color vision test are painless and productive.

Psychological Examinations

There are many types of psychological tests available today, each of which is designed for specific purposes. Psychological testing, however, rarely provides information of value in the diagnosis or management of the MS patient. Textbooks often characterize any mental changes noted in MS as euphoria (a sensation of well-being which persists despite the presence of obvious disabilities). Although euphoria is common, depression is equally so. In addition to mood disturbances, there may be subtle but important intellectual and cognitive deficits. Patients may complain of having difficulty performing their jobs or other intellectual tasks for reasons that cannot be detected by the usual methods of examination. Judiciously chosen psychological tests have revealed a high percentage of cognitive deficits in patients judged by even experienced physicians as being intellectually normal. Furthermore, there appears to be no correlation between the presence of such cognitive deficits and the presence or absence of other functional disability of the motor, sensory, or coordinative systems. Finally, because one of the commonest complaints of MS patients is lack of energy, psychological evaluation may be useful in differentiating this complaint from depression. The complaint of fatigability is often (erroneously) thought to be caused by depression in MS patients—the fatigue is real, although it is extremely difficult to ascribe it to weakness, stiffness, or any other physical causes.

Laboratory Examinations

Blood Tests

There are no abnormalities of the red blood cells, white blood cells, or platelets (cells involved in the clotting process) or of the chemical constituents of blood which provide any diagnostic clues in MS.

Immunological Tests

Many tests of immunological function (the body's system of defense against infection and other foreign substances) have been developed. None has any value in the diagnosis of MS at this time. The Levy test was recently shown by reliable investigators to be incapable of differentiating MS patients from others. Most immunological tests are not only highly specialized and not generally available, but their results vary considerably from one laboratory to the other, and their significance remains unclear.

Genetic Tests

The "histocompatibility system" consists of genetic material on a particular chromosome that controls the ability of a person to accept or reject tissue transplants (such as a kidney). Principally in Scandinavia and the United States, where large groups of MS patients have been studied, it has been demonstrated that specific types of this genetic material are present in a significant number of MS patients. From these studies has come the interesting suggestion that certain genetic factors may predispose individuals to acquiring MS. Studies have also been carried out in families in which more than one blood relative was affected by the disease. These studies have not provided any basis for the hope that examining the histocompatibility system in MS patients might reveal this predisposition. In one study the genetic characteristics of two siblings with MS in the same family were shown to be completely different, whereas in other families patients with MS and normal siblings shared identical genetic factors. Some medical centers have tried to use the information derived from such studies to help diagnose MS in individuals, but to no avail.

Cerebrospinal Fluid

For many years examination of the cerebrospinal fluid was considered absolutely necessary to confirm the diagnosis of MS. It was noted some years ago that many patients with MS had abnormal amounts of colloidal gold, and later that MS patients had an increased amount of gamma globulin in their cerebrospinal fluid. These findings indicated an immunological abnormality, and so the measurement of immunoglobulin G (IgG; a protein fraction of gamma globulin) became one of the standard diagnostic tests.

Unfortunately, an elevation of IgG is not specific for MS; it can be seen in a wide variety of other diseases, and so its elevation alone is not sufficient for establishing the diagnosis of MS. In many cases an incorrect diagnosis of MS has been based almost entirely on this laboratory observation in patients whose history and physical examination barely suggested MS. Furthermore, the reliability of this test varies considerably from hospital to hospital. In some research-oriented institutions it approaches a reliability of 65 to 70%, but in most others it is reliable only 40 to 50% of the time. However, it remains a useful confirmatory test in patients whose history and physical examination clearly indicate the diagnosis of MS.

The demonstration of a specific IgG (oligoclonal IgG bands) in cerebrospinal fluid has been reported as being positive in over 90% of patients with MS. This might be close to the ideal confirmatory laboratory test for MS. Unfortunately, a number of other conditions produce the same abnormality. When performing this test great attention must be paid to the details of the technique itself, so that its diagnostic value becomes highly questionable in all but a handful of institutions where the test is very carefully controlled. In those places it is an extraordinarily valuable confirmatory test for MS.

It is also possible now to measure the myelin basic protein (one of the breakdown products of myelin) in cerebrospinal fluid. This particular test is not very helpful in making the diagnosis as the material may be found in the cerebrospinal fluid in any illness in which myelin is destroyed. It is also of only minor value for determining the activity of the disease process for the same reason. Neither the elevation of IgG nor the presence of oligoclonal bands in the cerebrospinal fluid gives any indication about the severity of the disease or its degree of activity.

DIAGNOSIS OF AN EXACERBATION

Diagnosing a return of the symptoms of MS (that is, an exacerbation of the disease) remains critical to the management of a diagnosed patient. There are no definite clinical criteria by which we can judge that the disease process has been activated. Obviously, such a determination is of the utmost importance in instituting treatment and evaluation if it is effective.

New symptoms occur in only about one-fifth of patients with exacerbation of their disease. In other words, in four of five patients, symptoms noted when the disease flares are simply a recurrence of those experienced before. Because we now know that lesions do exist that never cause symptoms, new symptoms cannot necessarily be interpreted as evidence of the formation of new lesions; in fact, they may stem from lesions that have been "silent" up to now. The same thing is true of new signs.

In addition to the fact that a temperature elevation produces symptoms, other physiological disturbances (such as alterations in water and ion metabolism caused, for example, by vomiting and diarrhea) may similarly lead to the appearance of symptoms. Physical trauma, undue fatigue, and, most significantly, psychological stress may play an important role through yet unknown mechanisms in bringing out exacerbations. Because of this, hospitalization or even simple bed rest, and thus removal from the daily stress of work and home, may lead to the disappearance of often serious symptoms.

It bears repeating that exacerbations do not necessarily represent an aggravation of the disease. The rate of activity of the disease cannot be determined on the basis of clinical symptoms. In the same way, "improvement" brought about by certain forms of treatment may be due more to the enthusiasm of the dedicated investigator than to the treatment itself.

INFORMING THE PATIENT

Patients and their immediate families have every right to be told the diagnosis, especially the degree of certainty with which it has been established. The term "possible" MS should be avoided because it needlessly extends the period of anxiety for the patient. The use of euphemistic designations such as "demyelinating disease" or "inflammation of the white matter" is counterproductive. A patient should be assured that, contrary to popular belief, MS does not carry a uniformly poor prognosis. It should be pointed out that: (a) many MS patients have the disease in so mild a form that they never suffer any kind of disability because of it; (b) in others the dysfunction is mild and temporary; (c) the disease seems to be arrested or burned out in many patients; and (d) it is a minority of

MS patients who end up bedridden. A patient should be told not only to avoid heat but also how to take care of minor infections and prevent urinary tract infections. Such general supportive measures can be of great help in improving the long-term prognosis.

Patients with MS tend, as do others with slowly progressive or chronic illnesses, to seek other opinions and to search for new forms of treatment. If a patient is reluctant to accept the diagnosis of MS, it may be best to get a second opinion as quickly as possible from another well-known authority. All treatments should be carefully explained and discussed with the patient and family. Reassurance, sound information, and compassion must always be available for the MS patient.

CONCLUSION

It is often difficult to make a diagnosis of MS in its early stages. If the disease progresses, this becomes easy. The diagnosis is based on the demonstration—by the history, physical examination, and carefully chosen diagnostic procedures—that there are multiple lesions scattered throughout the white matter of the central nervous system. For many patients, laboratory procedures are not necessary but may be useful in confirming the clinical impression. Usually adequate confirmation can be obtained by the noninvasive, relatively inexpensive, simple procedure of measuring visual or other types of evoked responses. The CAT scan has limited usefulness in diagnosing this illness, and examination of the cerebrospinal fluid has been largely supplanted by other tests.

There is a natural tendency on the part of physicians to play it safe by ordering many tests which may in some way or another support the diagnosis. Engaging in such a diagnostic cascade, unfortunately at times demanded by the patient, is not only unwarranted but becomes extremely expensive and unpleasant, and is also potentially harmful.

4

Signs, Symptoms, and Course of the Disease

Labe Scheinberg

MS typically can be described as an unpredictable gait disorder whose onset is during early adult life. It is often associated with urinary and sexual symptoms. The disease is variable in its presentation, manifestations, and course.

The disease may begin at almost any age. There have been proved cases with an onset during early childhood and some that occurred in the latter part of the sixth decade of life, but 90% of the cases begin in individuals between the ages of 15 and 50 years. The average age of onset is about 30 years.

There is a definite sex predilection, with the majority of cases occurring in females. Various studies have reported that 55 to 80% of the patients are women.

The geographic and racial distribution of the disease is interesting. Generally it occurs two or three times more often in northern latitudes; that is, it is more prevalent in temperate zones than in tropical or subtropical regions. These areas of increased prevalence are referred to as high-risk zones and the others as low-risk zones. Certain countries (Japan, for example), though in the same latitude as the northern United States, have a very low incidence. The reasons for these variations are not clear and probably have something to do with both environmental and genetic factors. Certain races or ethnic groups other than the Japanese have an unusually low incidence even though they reside in high-risk zones (for example, gypsies and Inuits), and certain locales (for example, the Shetland Islands) have an unusually high prevalence.

If one moves from a low-risk zone to a high-risk zone early in life (usually at less than 15 years of age), the individual has the same chance of getting MS as if he had been born in the high-risk zone. On the other hand, if the individual moves later in life to a high-risk zone, the risk is the same as if he had remained in the zone of origin. This has led many to conclude that MS is a disease with an onset during childhood but one that may not manifest for many years. Moreover, it is obvious that once the disease has appeared, it is of little or no benefit to move to low-risk zones. It is quite apparent that both genetic and environmental factors play a role in the cause and development of MS (see Chapter 2).

The initial and later symptoms of MS are of four general types: motor (movement) 35%, sensory (touch) 35%, visual 20%, and other (bladder, bowel, mental, etc.) 10%.

Symptoms are subjective complaints (for example, blurred vision, numbness, or weakness). Signs are objective changes observed by the physician (for example, decreased sensation or reflex abnormalities). Symptoms and signs collectively are referred to as "findings."

MOTOR SYMPTOMS

Weakness

Most often one or both legs are affected by MS, but the arms or half the face may be involved as well. This may initially be experienced as a "heaviness" or easy fatigue after walking short distances. It is called "paraparesis" if the legs are involved and "quadriparesis" if all extremities are involved. Total paralysis is called paraplegia (legs) or quadriplegia (all limbs) and is rare in MS.

Spasticity

Spasticity usually manifests in the legs by a feeling of stiffness or tightness, and in severe cases it may be characterized by involuntary spontaneous jerking movements of the legs. Often with spasticity of the legs, the patient will notice shaking or jerking of the leg when the toe is placed on the floor and the knee is flexed. This is a sign of spasticity called "clonus." If one relaxes fully, it may be difficult for the examiner to move the spastic extremity easily.

Ataxia

Ataxia generally refers to difficulty in walking caused by a loss of balance or incoordination of the legs. The individual will be unable to walk—as when trying to "tandem gait" (walking heel to toe on a line); in more severe cases he will stagger and sway from side to side. In very severe cases the individual will be unable to walk even though the legs are strong; he may even sway or his head will bob when he is sitting unsupported.

In the upper extremities there may be loss of coordination during rapid, fine motor acts, or he may experience tremors when attempting to perform such tests as touching the finger to the nose (intention tremor). Rarely, involuntary movements may occur while the arm or leg are at rest.

Gait disorders varying from an inability to walk the usual distance to an inability to walk at all are the principal problems of patients with MS. This may be a result of any combination of the aforementioned: weakness, spasticity, or ataxia combined with easy fatigibility, which is discussed later.

One constellation of symptoms, called "spastic paraparesis of middle age," is a common presentation of the spinal form of MS. It appears during the fourth or fifth decade of life. It is usually insidiously progressive, and many of these patients are believed to have arthritis of the spine or tumors pressing on the cord. However, if there is no pain or other sensory complaints or findings, it is much more likely due to MS. Moreover, early bladder and sexual complaints indicate that MS is the cause. Nonetheless, many such patients have myelograms performed at least once to rule out the diagnosis of spinal cord compression by tumor or arthritis.

Speech Disorder

Speech disorder is a motor symptom seen in MS that was described as part of "Charcot's triad" in the original clinical description of MS along with "intention tremor" and nystagmus (a jerking movement of the eyes). The patient knows what he wants to say and can understand everything but has difficulty in articulation. Scanning speech (in which the syllables seem to be separated by pauses), described originally by Charcot, is an example of ataxic dysarthria. Other types of articulation disorders, such as spastic dysarthria (in which imprecise consonants, slow rate, low pitch, and harsh voice quality) and mixed dysarthrias, are more common in MS. Language problems (called "aphasias") are almost never seen in MS.

SENSORY SYMPTOMS

Numbness

Tingling, pins-and-needles, or feelings of tightness (medical term—"paresthesias") in one or more extremity or part of the body or face is a common symptom at the beginning or during the course of MS. It may begin in a hand or foot and progress until it involves the lower half or entire one-half of the body. It may occur as a tight band or girdle sensation around the trunk. Generally sensory symptoms tend to clear within a few months.

Pain

Sharp, brief pain following the course of a nerve root (medical term—"dermatome") is seen in some patients. Most often it involves the face, where it is called "trigeminal neuralgia," but other parts of the body may be involved. Burning pains or cold sensations of longer duration are also seen.

Passively bending the neck forward may produce brief tingling, electric-like sensations down the back, arms, or legs. This phenomenon is characteristic of MS and has been given the name "Lhermitte's sign."

Visual Symptoms

Blurred vision is a common symptom at the beginning or during the course of MS. It may appear within a few hours or days and usually involves one eye. The central vision is usually impaired so that only large objects or movements can be seen. It may be accompanied by some pain or tenderness in the eye, and in rare cases the other eye may be involved a few days or weeks later. This is called "optic or retrobulbar neuritis." About two-thirds improve or clear completely within a few months. Complete visual loss is very rare.

When one sees blurred vision in one eye in a young adult, major diagnostic problems are raised. Depending on the length of time varied groups of patients with this presentation are followed, the complete picture of MS will occur in 15 to 80% of cases. On average about 40% of patients will develop other signs of MS within 15 years, but some may live a full life without additional problems. There are very few other causes of optic neuritis in the young adult, and many doctors would consider such an episode to be a single attack of benign MS.

Double vision (medical term—"diplopia") is noted by some patients when they look in a certain direction; they may report this at the beginning or during the course of the disease. It disappears when one eye is closed. This is a result of weakness of one or more eye muscles and may be eliminated by closing either eye. Occasionally objects will appear to jump or move in the field of vision. These symptoms usually clear within weeks or months.

Other Symptoms

Dizziness (medical term—"vertigo") is a symptom seen in MS. The patient may describe the feeling of turning or spinning, and it is often accompanied by nausea or vomiting. This symptom usually clears within a few days or weeks.

Deafness is a less common symptom of MS and often is detected only on audiometric testing. Tinnitus (ringing in the ears) is a very rare symptom of MS.

Urinary symptoms are very common sometime during the course of MS and may even be the presenting complaints. These may be urgency to urinate, frequency of urination with getting up at night (nocturia), inability to urinate (retention), or loss of control (incontinence). A secondary common complication is urinary tract infection manifested by painful urination or burning (dysuria), frequency, urgency, fever, and lower abdominal or back pain. The urine may be cloudy and foul-smelling. These are discussed further, along with bowel problems, in Chapter 10.

Bowel problems are less common than bladder problems. They are usually associated with bladder disorders and the fluid restriction practiced by many patients in an effort to control incontinence and other urinary problems. Constipation is the most common symptom, but loss of control is also seen infrequently.

Sexual problems are common in both sexes. Loss of sexual drive is common with impotence of varying degree in the male, and it may be caused by an inability to achieve or maintain an erection or to ejaculate. Psychological or emotional disorders produce similar complaints and obviously play some role in the MS person. In the female, failure to achieve a climax (anorgasmy) or change in sexual satisfaction is common. The ability to become pregnant is not usually involved. Sexual problems may be secondary to motor symptoms (such as weakness or spasticity) or a loss of sensation in the genital region, or it may occur independently. Sexual and bowel problems are often associated, as nerve centers controlling these functions are in the same location in the spinal cord.

Energy problems, including a lack of energy, easy fatigability, tiredness, or listlessness, are common problems seen in MS patients even in the absence of other motor complaints. The MS person may not have the endurance to perform more than a few hours' work, and the condition is aggravated by humid and warm environments. This may cause one to confuse these complaints with those due to anxiety or depression, but the exact cause is a mystery. These problems tend to clear after many months.

Mental symptoms do affect these individuals. Characteristically, the MS person has been stereotyped as cheerful (medical term—

"euphoric"), but the majority show depression and anxiety early in the course due to difficulty adapting to the disability and fear for the future. Later, mental symptoms may appear with irritability, some memory loss, forgetfulness, and even confusion and disorientation late in the course in about 25% of cases. Early intellectual deterioration may appear rarely in the so-called cerebral form of the disease, where there are extensive lesions in the central myelin of the parts of the brain associated with mental functioning.

Not infrequently, mental symptoms associated with tiredness or listlessness may be the presenting complaint without any objective findings. This may lead to the erroneous diagnosis of psychoneurosis or even more severe psychiatric disorder.

After a period of more than 20 years of illness, about 25% of patients show significant mental changes, and, rarely, severe dementia is also seen.

Certain symptoms (such as seizures, loss of consciousness, headache, and language disturbances) are very rare in MS. The presence and persistence of these symptoms should lead to further investigation.

COURSE

The course of MS is unpredictable. The average life expectancy after onset is about 35 years. Some rare cases follow a rapidly progressive course to death within a few months, but the average patient may expect to live 90% or more of their expected life span.

The patterns of the disease usually seen are: (a) *Benign form*, with few, mild early attacks (medical term—"exacerbations") and complete or nearly complete clearing (medical term—"remissions"). The patient has a normal life expectancy and minimal or no disability. About 20% of cases fall into this category. (b) *Exacerbating-remitting form*, with more frequent, early attacks and less complete clearing but showing long periods of stability. Some degree of disability is usually present. About 25% of cases follow this pattern. (c) *Chronic-relapsing form*, with fewer and less-complete remissions after attacks. The disability is cumulative and greater than seen in the previous forms. The course may run for many years and then plateau with moderate to severe disability. About 40% of cases are of this type. (d) *Chronic-progressive form*, which is similar to the previous form except the onset is more insidious, and the course is slowly progressive without remissions. About 15% of all cases follow this pattern.

An *exacerbation*, or attack, is defined as an acute appearance of new symptoms or worsening of old symptoms which lasts at least 24 hours. Sometimes this occurs in association with acute fevers, usually due to urinary tract infections, and it is called a "pseudoexacerbation."

A *remission* is a total or more often partial clearing of symptoms and signs which lasts more than 24 hours. When the patient's condition is stable for a long period (months or years), it is called a "remission" also, or "plateau." To be significant, a remission should last at least 1 month.

When severe disability is produced by the MS itself (without skin or joint contracture complications), it is a result of (a) severe weakness with or without spasticity; (b) severe incoordination; (c) loss of bladder and bowel control; or rarely (d) dementia. Visual loss and sensory disturbances are rarely a cause of disability.

Although it is difficult from the initial symptom to predict what is going to happen to the individual case, there are some indications from the presentation of the disease that help predict its future course. As a general rule, when the patient presents with only an abrupt onset of sensory symptoms or blurred vision which clears completely, one can often predict a less severe course. If motor symptoms (such as weakness or incoordination) present initially and progress slowly, the result is often greater disability. There are many exceptions, and during the first few years of the disease many almost miraculous remissions occur spontaneously or coincidental to some treatment. After 5 years the remissions are less frequent, and often incomplete recovery is seen.

After the first 5 years, one can often predict if the course will be benign or otherwise, and if it is progressing to disability. One can then frequently predict if the disability will be due to spastic weakness of the extremities or incoordination. Treatment for spasticity is usually effective, and bladder symptoms respond well to medical intervention. However, weakness, incoordination, and the rarely seen mental deterioration are unresponsive to most if not all treatments. Any improvements seen in these disabilities are usually spontaneous or coincidental.

MS with an onset after age 35 is usually characterized by a slow, progressive weakness of the legs often accompanied by bladder and sexual problems. In most cases these patients need aids for ambulation but do not become confined to a wheelchair.

MS itself is almost never a cause of death. When the disease does shorten the life span, it is a result of intercurrent infection involving either the lungs (pneumonia), urinary tract (pyelonephritis or cystitis), or skin (pressure sores, or decubiti). The appearance of significant urinary complaints and infections, intractable spasticity, joint contractures, and pressure sores with infection are indications of the late stages of MS and should be prevented by good medical-nursing care whenever possible. As a result of these measures, the life expectancy of the patient with MS has been increased by 10 years since the 1950s.

PRECIPITATING AND AGGRAVATING FACTORS

There has been a great deal of speculation over the years as to the course of a new attack. Perhaps the most frequent factor cited by patients and families is emotional stress and psychological trauma. It is difficult to prove or disprove the role of emotions in the precipitation of attacks or cause of progression, as, conversely, the sudden appearance of new symptoms or progression is a cause of emotional distress.

In summary, MS is an unpredictable disease of the nervous system which manifests primarily by disorders in mobility. It is associated with a variety of other primary and secondary symptoms and complications. In general it is compatible with a long and productive life.

5

Drug Therapy

Labe Scheinberg and Barbara S. Giesser

The goals of therapy of any disease are to prevent the initial occurrence (prophylactic treatment), to arrest the progress of the disease and prevent future attacks (curative treatment), to repair the damaged tissues and restore them to normal function (restorative treatment), to treat symptoms, to prevent and relieve complications (symptomatic treatment), and to help the patient to adjust to the disability and achieve as much function as possible with the remaining normal tissues or parts (rehabilitative therapy).

The cause of MS is not known. Moreover, one can only conjecture as to the mechanism of tissue damage which produces the impairment. Finally, it is the nature of the tissues of the central nervous system to regenerate poorly, if at all, after severe damage. Considering these factors, the treatment of MS is very frustrating and disappointing.

At present there is little or probably no treatment that will prevent the initial or future attacks of MS. Although there is excellent prophylactic treatment in many infectious diseases (for example, poliomyelitis, smallpox, measles), there is nothing available for MS because no virus or other infectious agent has been identified. Recently MS was reported theoretically to be related to distemper in dogs, and it has been suggested that eradication of distemper by immunizing dogs would reduce or eliminate MS. However, this is speculative and unproved. It also does little or nothing to help MS patients who already have significant damage and disability.

There are no known curative therapies that will arrest the course of MS or even alter the natural history of attacks and remissions or halt progression. Many things have been employed over the last

45

century, and many new methods of treatment are undergoing clinical testing, but it is highly debatable if anything will significantly change the pattern of the disease at this time. It has been reported that certain hormones [for example, cortisone or adrenocorticotropic hormone (ACTH, or corticotropin)] shorten an individual attack, but do not prevent future attacks and probably have little or no effect on the long-term functioning of the patient. Other drugs and treatments have produced less evidence of benefit, and many reported "cures" or ameliorations are probably coincidental to the natural fluctuations of the disease.

Many symptoms and signs do clear partially, or even completely, following an attack. It is believed that these partial or complete remissions are due to the clearing of inflammation and edema in the acute lesions. In large and more severe lesions, the myelin at the center of the lesion, or plaque, may be severely damaged, and so only partial or possibly no remission occurs. With subsequent attacks, the lesions, or plaques, enlarge and the deficit increases, which explains why early in the course of MS any treatments are effective and later most are ineffective.

Once there is a large plaque, or lesion, in the central myelin (tissue surrounding the nerves) with sclerosis (scarring), one must hope that there is some treatment that will restore or repair the damaged myelin and/or improve nerve conduction through the damaged area. Unfortunately, at present there is no restorative therapy which will repair the damage or improve conduction in the region of the plaque.

Today symptomatic and rehabilitative therapy are the most effective approaches available. One may use drugs effectively to relieve certain symptoms (such as spasticity or pain) which are a direct result of the plaques (lesions) in the myelin of the central nervous system. Symptoms such as weakness, spasticity, incoordination, pain, numbness, urinary urgency, incontinence, retention, blurred vision, and others are "primary symptoms" which are related to plaques in specific locations. Other symptoms, such as urinary tract infections (cystitis), bed sores (decubiti), and contractures of joints are a result of the primary symptoms and should be called "secondary symptoms." These are generally responsive to drug, surgical, or physical therapies and are discussed in detail later. Finally, there are symptoms and other developments which are a result of the primary and secondary symptoms; these should be called "tertiary symptoms" and include such problems as depression, marital problems, loss of employment, etc. These tertiary symptoms, or problems, are often amenable to psychosocial interventions such as counseling and job modification. These approaches are discussed extensively in later chapters.

These points of view have been stated eloquently by Dr. Tore Broman, a prominent Swedish neurologist who has had extensive experience in the management of MS. He stated:

> Many attempts have been made to find a causal and preventive treatment for multiple sclerosis, but they have all failed and are, therefore, rather illustrative of empirical trials based on more or less vaguely founded working hypotheses. This fact led to one or two opposite prejudicial attitudes, which were more common earlier, but still are sadly prevalent. One of these represents the nihilistic attitude towards any kind of measure for helping the patients: 'I am sorry, but there is no treatment, so I cannot help you.' And the other one is the optimistic and magical belief in having found out the key method for curing the disease: 'Come to me, I have elaborated a new method to treat multiple sclerosis and I have already cured hundreds of patients.' There is today only one attitude to the multiple sclerosis patients worthy of a neurologist and that is: 'I cannot cure your disease, but it may run a benign course and anyhow I will try to help you, because much can be done to make life easier for you.'

In order to accomplish these goals, treatment can be divided into four general categories:

1. Pharmacological—use of drugs.
2. Surgical—use of such surgical measures as cutting nerves or tendons, skin grafts, etc.
3. Physical—use of exercises, massage, stretching, heat, cold, or electrical stimulation.
4. Psychological—use of counseling or other psychiatric treatment.

An excellent reference to most of the therapies currently being employed is the book, *Therapeutic Claims in Multiple Sclerosis*, published under the auspices of the International Federation of Multiple Sclerosis Societies. It may be purchased from the National Multiple Sclerosis Society, 205 East 42 Street, New York, N.Y. 10017. The book reviews about 120 treatments, giving the rationales, benefits, and risks for each. It will be updated as new treatments are developed or the use of experimental ones is proved or disproved. This book is highly recommended and will even counter the sometimes insistent advice of well-meaning family and friends.

GENERAL GUIDELINES IN MANAGEMENT

It is important to state some general guidelines in the management prior to discussion of specific treatments. These have been learned by experience with large numbers of patients and families.

1. The patient and significant others should be informed of the diagnosis when the neurologist or other competent physician is certain of it. The diagnosis should be "multiple sclerosis," a term most people know, and not such terms as "demyelinating disease," "chronic virus infections of the nervous system," "allergy of the nervous system," "encephalomyelitis," etc.

When patients are not informed at the time the diagnosis is established but learn of it later, they may become angry at the initial physician and not trust him. Often patients are relieved to learn the diagnosis because they had suspected a more serious condition or believed that they had a psychological disorder. Almost all patients can accept the diagnosis and cope with it. It is essential to reveal the diagnosis so that patients and families can plan for the future, avail themselves of the various services and benefits that are available to MS patients, and embark on a sound therapeutic regimen. The diagnosis should be discussed fully along with a presentation of current knowledge of the disease. It should not be unduly optimistic or pessimistic as the future course cannot be predicted.

2. The patient should be given a return appointment and not told, "There's no cure, so just go home and learn to live with it." The

frequency of return visits depends on the severity, rate of progression, complications, and other factors. The return visits are useful for detecting and treating new findings of MS and complications, for counseling the patient and family, and for discussing new developments in treatment and research.

3. The patient should be managed when necessary by a team of health professionals consisting of neurologists, physiatrists, psychiatrists, urologists, internists, nurses, physical therapists, occupational therapists, social workers, rehabilitation counselors, and psychologists. Few diseases have as many varied long-term ramifications, and few require the services of so many professionals at some time or other during their course. Few solo practitioners are prepared to deal with so complex a disease during its long course. Not all cases require these services, but patients and families should be aware of the possibilities should the need ever arise.

4. The patient should participate actively in his management. This disease, as so many others, makes the patient feel that he has lost control, and so he should be encouraged to participate in the adjustment of certain drugs, management of the bladder, rehabilitation, diet, and physical therapy. Most therapeutic decisions are somewhat empirical, and the patient can effectively participate. When the patient does not follow instructions or embarks on a treatment course not recommended by the physician, later recriminations should be avoided. With the exception of surgery, unproved treatments often do not cause the disease to worsen but may incur unnecessary expense and, later, disappointment.

5. The patient should fully discuss any new treatments and be warned about unwarranted optimism; over the decades most "cures" have not withstood the test of time and have often benefited only the therapists.

In this presentation of drug management, only those agents which we generally employ are discussed. There are many schedules for any drug, but only those we have found to be easily followed and of benefit are presented. Occasionally some other drugs or routes of administration are discussed briefly as these may be used by other physicians.

DRUG THERAPY OF PRIMARY SYMPTOMS

The major primary symptoms of MS are motor disabilities (weakness, stiffness or spasticity, incoordination, loss of balance, gait difficulties, and tremors). Weakness and other motor symptoms, if seen as part of an acute attack, may respond to short-term antiinflammatory agents, such as ACTH (adrenocorticotropic hormone, or corticotropin), adrenal corticosteroids, and synthetic glucocorticoids (prednisone). These drugs are administered for brief periods, almost never more than 1 month at a time. Long-term or chronic use is not recommended. The drug may be taken again for brief periods if there is a recurrence or a new attack, but the effect is often less in each subsequent bout. Our method is to give either ACTH or prednisone in the following manner as we have found it to be simpler, to be less costly, and to have fewer side effects while offering as great a benefit as other methods. Moreover, these methods generally do not require hospital care, and injections may be given by a visiting nurse or other competent individual.

Prednisone, 40 milligrams (mg) in divided dosage (10 mg four times a day after food ingestion) taken on alternate days for 1 month, seems to be as effective as other regimens, and the schedule is simple with few complications.

Prednisone, adrenal corticosteroids, and synthetic glucocorticoids have been taken by other routes (intravenous, intramuscular, intraspinal, or intrathecal) but do not seem to be any more effective and may be more hazardous and costly. In fact, although some doctors use intraspinal or intrathecal injections, most consider it to be too hazardous for intravenous or intramuscular injection of a sustained-released repository gel (Acthar or Corticotrophin Gel). It is our practice to give the gel form intramuscularly, 80 units daily for 5 days and then 40 units daily for 5 days. This seems to be as effective as when it is given by the intravenous route, and it does not require hospitalization or confinement to bed for any period.

Again, there is little proof that ACTH and adrenal corticosteroids are very effective except for short-term use to reduce the severity of individual acute attacks. In fact, adrenal corticosteroids have never been tested properly for this disease, and their use has been based on the results of ACTH studies. It has even been stated that if two large groups of MS patients were using ACTH and adrenal corticosteroids for acute attacks (in one group) or nothing (in the other group), the final disability in the two groups would be identical after 10 to 20 years. There is certainly no basis for long-term chronic use of either of these agents.

The complications of therapy with these agents are minimal with short-term use. They include transiently generalized puffiness, weight gain, psychosis, peptic ulcer, general infections, and acne. With long-term daily therapy, there is in addition the risk of abnormalities in blood levels of sodium and potassium, bone softening with fractures, cataracts, hypertension, diabetes, and adrenal exhaustion.

In conclusion, short-term therapy with ACTH or adrenal corticosteroids carries little risk and seems to be of value in reducing the severity of an individual bout, whereas long-term use does not appear to alter the course and is hazardous.

Spasticity is a motor symptom that can be disabling and even painful. It may cause difficulty in walking, restrict the range of motion of the extremities, and result in painful muscle spasms. If not properly managed it may result in urinary complications, contractures of the joints, and eventually pressure sores (decubitus ulcers). Three agents have been recommended for controlling spasticity: baclofen (Lioresal), diazepam (Valium), and dantrolene sodium (Dantrium). We employ only baclofen. Diazepam seems to be less effective, produces excessive sedation, and even causes psychic and physical dependence; and dantrolene sodium produces nausea, diarrhea, and carries a long-term risk of liver damage and pleural effusions (fluid collection in the chest).

The recommended dose of baclofen is from 15 mg (1½ tablets) daily to 80 mg (eight tablets) daily given in three or four doses. Occasionally a higher dose must be taken to alleviate severe spasticity; this may be as much as 150 mg a day, even though the Federal Drug Administration (FDA) recommends a maximum of 80 mg a day. Initially, some patients complain of drowsiness, but this is transitory. Others complain of loss of appetite and nausea, both of which can be avoided by taking the drug after meals. More important, many patients report increased sensation of weakness of the legs and greater gait difficulties with this drug. This is due to a reduction of spasticity, making the weakness already present more apparent. Because the dividing line between spasticity and weakness is indistinct, we often advise patients to adjust the dose themselves from time to time. If one takes too much, the legs are excessively flaccid, or "rubbery," and the dose should be reduced. A return to the previous level of spasticity occurs within hours after changing the dose. If one takes an insufficient dose, the legs feel too spastic, or "tight," and the dose should be increased.

Withdrawal from the drug should be done gradually, over a few days, as transient seizures and hallucinations have been reported, although rarely.

Tremor, loss of coordination, ataxia, and loss of balance with gait difficulties are troublesome and disabling symptoms, and unfortunately are resistant to any known drugs. Some have tried propranolol (Inderal) to relieve tremor, but we have found this agent to have no benefit even at very high dosage. The management of tremor and related symptoms requires other therapeutic measures, which are also minimally effective.

Speech disorders, another motor symptom, do not respond to any currently available drug. Fortunately, they are rarely disabling.

Sensory symptoms (such as numbness, tingling, pins-and-needles, and pain) are common but usually not disabling or permanent. When the pain is severe, it should be treated with carbamazepine (Tegretol®). Phenytoin (Dilantin®) and amitriptyline (Elavil® and others) are often useful for painful numbness or tingling. The dose is similar to that employed in other neurological pain disorders: 200 to 1,600 mg daily (one to eight tablets) given in divided doses (two to four times a day). This is usually effective with minimal side effects (drowsiness, loss of appetite, and nausea). The patients should be followed regularly by their physician, who should closely monitor the effects of the drug.

Other sensory symptoms (such as visual symptoms) also do not cause significant disability, and we rarely use any drugs in these cases. Occasionally, one may employ ACTH or adrenal corticosteroids for severe visual symptoms due to inflammation of the optic nerve. These symptoms are usually transient and in most cases clear spontaneously within 2 to 3 months or less. Vertigo is usually transitory and may be treated with meclazine hydrochloride (Antivert or Bonine).

Urinary symptoms are common, and it is important to manage them carefully. One of the major approaches to this is drug therapy in conjunction with other measures (Chapter 10).

The use of certain drugs to control muscle contractions of the urinary bladder is important when the patient complains of primary urinary symptoms (urgency, frequency, incontinence, and urinary retention). These drugs are called anticholinergics or antispasmodics and include a number of preparations. The most frequently employed are propantheline bromide (Pro-Banthine and other generic preparations), dicyclomine hydrochloride (Bentyl and other generic preparations), flavoxate hydrochloride (Urispas), hyoscymine (Cystospaz), and oxybutynin chloride (Ditropan). All of these must be prescribed by a physician and the dosage monitored for the patient and adjusted if necessary at varying times in the course of the illness. Although there is no conclusive evidence that one anticholinergic agent is superior to another, we have found that patients become less responsive to one after a period of time and then respond to another.

All have the common side effects of this class of drugs: dryness of the mouth, constipation, drowsiness, photophobia (sensitivity to light), and blurred vision. Sometimes it is necessary to accept these side effects in order to achieve the benefits for the bladder. In some cases, complete transient paralysis of the urinary detrusor muscle occurs or may even be the desired goal to control symptoms. This is discussed later in conjunction with intermittent catheterization.

Some members of another class of drugs, the tricyclic antidepressants, are often useful in the management of uncontrollable urinary muscle contractions. One drug especially, imipramine (Tofranil and other generic preparations), is often used. It has the same side effects as the anticholinergic drugs but is advantageous in that it may be administered once a day because of its long duration of action; it also produces some antidepressant action, which is desirable for some patients.

Another class of drugs—the alpha-adrenergic blocking agents, which act on the autonomic nervous system—has also been tried. One drug, phenoxybenzamine (Dibenzyline) is believed by some physicians to be of use in relaxing the bladder muscle in certain cases. It is said to be useful in relaxing the sphincter muscle of the bladder to relieve functional obstruction to urinary outflow. Its major side effect is orthostatic hypotension (it lowers the blood pressure when the patient is standing).

Infections are common and should be treated with specific antibiotics. The infecting organism should be identified and the specific antibiotic to combat it determined. Sometimes long-term prophylaxis to urinary tract infection is attempted by the use of nitrofurantoin (Macrodantin or Furadantin), nalidixic acid (Negram), sulfonamides (Gantrisin or Gantanol), or a sulfonamide mixed with another drug (Bactrim or Septra). Drugs for urinary tract infection should be administered only under careful medical supervision.

Other drugs used to prevent urinary tract infection are methenamine hippurate (Hiprex or Urex) and methenamine mandelate (Mandelamine). These may be given for long periods of time at a dose of 2.0 grams (g) daily in divided dosage for the methenamine hippurate or 4.0 g in divided dosage for the methenamine mandelate). These drugs are effective as urinary tract antiseptics only in an acidic urine. They are therefore given in conjunction with vitamin C (ascorbic acid) 4.0 g daily in divided dosage (Chapter 10).

DISCUSSION

The list of drugs that have been and are currently used for MS is almost endless. Only those which seem to give some benefit and which have few or no side effects are discussed. Although no drug seems to significantly alter the long-term course of MS, many give symptomatic relief.

One area of major controversy is the use of immunosuppressive agents—azathioprine (Imuran), cyclophosphamide (Cytoxan), and others—in the long-term management of MS. These agents suppress activity of the immune system of the body and have a theoretical basis for use. They are currently undergoing clinical trials and cannot yet be said to definitely benefit the patient. Moreover, these drugs present serious risks to the patient (such as bone marrow suppression, concurrent infection, loss of hair, gastrointestinal disturbance, cancer, and birth defects). The use of these drugs should be limited at present.

6

Treatment with Diet

James Q. Simmons

A frequent question posed by those with MS is: Can I eat some special things that will make me well? Is there a diet that will help my MS? The immediate answer of course is that many diets for MS, often claiming cures, have in past years been promoted by doctors and others. Many theories have been advanced to justify diets of various sorts: For example, "The illness is allergic in nature, so eliminate foods to which many are sensitive." "There are deficiencies of minerals, vitamins, or hormones." "There is too much fat in the diet—or perhaps too little; therefore fatty foods in the diet must be reduced, changed in content, or even, as thought at one time, increased in the diet!"

The protein of wheat or rye flour, called gluten, was said to be the cause of MS just as it is the cause of a distressing intestinal condition in infants and children. Another doctor thought that modern foods produced by artificial fertilizer (not by good dependable manure) had all the life removed by excessive processing and overcooking. The answer—eat your food raw!

Several other proposals have appeared. You need manganese— buckwheat cakes are full of manganese—eat them daily. And do not forget sprouted grain—it is full of the very essence of new life and procreated growth for all the body tissues. Vitamins and minerals in very high dosage are sometimes prescribed.

Attempts to find consistent deficiencies in blood plasma fats of several kinds have had ambiguous results. The differences between those with MS and normal individuals have been minor. Conclusions reached were that findings can be interpreted to support the view that "the plasma lipid changes are secondary to multiple sclerosis and do not reflect any primary inherent lipid abnormality."

RECOMMENDED DIETS

Here are some of the recommended diets.

Allergen-Free Diet

Earliest among the diets proposed was the allergen-free diet. To be eliminated were the foods most frequently found to cause problems: milk, butter, eggs, citrus fruits, chocolate, tomatoes, cucumbers, and cabbage. These foods are sometimes incriminated in gastric distress, skin eruptions, asthma, or colitis. Whereas a disturbance of the immune system has been theorized to cause MS, the term did not apply to these allergic ills but to autoimmunity (sensitivity and reaction to one's own body tissue). A few doctors continue to seek an allergic basis for MS. Principal among them today is Arthur L. Kaslow of Santa Barbara, California. He determines "metabolic blockades and pathologic intolerances" to specific foods through his carbohydrate tolerance test. Those he treats are trained to recognize their own food intolerances. He combines with this a modification of acupuncture, using electrical point stimulators instead of acupuncture needles. He also treats those coming to him with a high level of concerned care.

Low-Fat Diet

Dr. Roy L. Swank of Oregon University Medical Center in Portland has, for some 30 years, urged a diet of foods containing the equivalent of 7 teaspoons of fat a day—the amount required by everyone for good health maintenance. Four teaspoons should be unsaturated fatty acid fats (found in seafood, nuts, and vegetables), and three teaspoons may be from animal foods. Swank has written a text that has had several editions containing recipes, menus, and his philosophy and advice. His is an excellent diet suitable for the healthy average man. He claims that those using his diet have fewer periods of worsening and better general health.

Raw Food Diet

Dr. Joseph Evers of Hachen, West Germany, gave his patients a raw food diet. He believed that modern food production and processing could not be trusted—so we must eat our food raw. I had driven 200 miles to visit him and we had stopped at the local Gasthaus for a plentiful breakfast only to be introduced a few minutes later to a giant table bowed down with a burden of raw root vegetables, sprouted grain, whole wheat bread, cheese, raw milk, raw eggs, butter, honey, and raw ham. He forbade salads, rhubarb, cauliflower, asparagus, sugar, salt, mustard, vinegar, and pepper.

Afterward we climbed a mountainside where a hospital was being built for the use of Evers who had brought 15,000 MS patients and their families to this small town. When finished, the health officials said "You now have a fine place to test your diet. Give every other patient your diet and a good German diet to the others." Evers vehemently avowed, "The only way to test the Evers diet is to give it to everyone." After his death in 1977 one of his two doctor sons, Paul Evers, continued to dispense his raw food practice at a nearby clinic in Sundern-Langscheid. He has an added recommendation—unsaturated fatty acid fats.

Gluten-Free Diet

Dr. R. Shatin of Melbourne, Australia, compared geographic areas where wheat, rye, and other grains containing a protein called gluten are grown with the prevalence rates in these areas for MS. He found high rates of MS in the grain-growing regions and low rates where rice and corn were grown and consumed. Shatin cited some studies on known disease conditions due to gluten and decided that MS could be a pathologic expression of gluten sensitivity.

MacDougall Diet

In 1974, letters—26,000 in the first wave—swarmed into the crowded confines of our Department of Medical Programs of the National Multiple Sclerosis Society. Roger MacDougall, a once successful Hollywood writer, had appeared in the pages of the *In-*

quirer, cane aloft and feet flying. He had found a diet which cured him of his MS. He had, he said, come upon it after years of study. It appeared to be a combination of things that had for years been recommended by others. It contained little fat and was gluten-free, with higher vitamin and mineral supplements and a few other things. It was the biggest event in the MS diet kingdom. We hired a firm to send out our MacDougall memorandum to the thousands who were excited by a prospect of help for their MS. He prohibits refined sugar, cream, and butter and offered margarine made from seed oils. Three times daily one took the vitamins and minerals in moderately high dosage.

High Manganese Diet

Dr. Robert M. Hill, a one-time biochemistry professor at the University of Colorado Medical Center in Denver, and a nephew with MS, who had worked in Hill's laboratories and his nutritional studies, demonstrated a manganese deficiency in MS patients. Correction he said was simple—eat buckwheat cakes each day—a superior source of the mineral. Can you think of a more pleasant cure?

High Vitamin Dosage

Dr. Frederick Klenner of North Carolina gives exceptionally high doses of all the vitamins, a variety of minerals, and other substances to MS patients. He adds a high protein diet and forbids smoking. He states that his treatment must often be followed for a number of years to be effective. He is an intelligent and able biochemist from Duke and has a stated reason for each substance he recommends.

Balanced Diet

The American public is given more dietary information than any people in the world. The public press carries articles by nutritionists. The Department of Agriculture, as part of the School Lunch Program, distributes pamphlets on a well-balanced diet. The Departments of Agriculture of each state provide booklets. Most can be obtained either free or for a few cents.

Comment

The Society can recommend at this time only the diet approved by scientific nutritionists. Its elements are discussed below.

GENERAL HEALTH

It may appear ludicrous when speaking of someone with MS to emphasize maintenance of a high level of general health. He has MS! But one with MS can be in good health or in poor health. One may fail to lead a healthy, reasonably active life and be in poor general health. He may neglect oral and general hygiene, proper nutrition, elimination, and insistence on living as fully as possible. He may become dependent. As for the diet, it should contain in balanced proportion each of the food groups: meat, vegetable–fruit, milk, and bread–cereal groups.

ESSENTIAL FOOD ELEMENTS

Food required for good health are found in these groups: protein, carbohydrates, fats, minerals, vitamins, and water. No *single* food gives every element or quantity needed. Different groups provide the entire spectrum of needs to work as a team for a good mix of all that is necessary for vigorous health.

To determine the quantity of food needed, we use the unit of food energy produced by foods used in the body—the *calorie*. One gram of protein or carbohydrate contains 4.5 calories; fat contains a troublesome 9 calories. The food types needed for good body function depend on the level of physical activity. Table 1 shows examples of this difference in food required with differences in activity level. If food is taken in excess of the requirements of these activities, there is fat build-up and obesity. Overweight places a strain on muscles and the heart, and body efficiency suffers.

Protein

Important building blocks for tissue repair are derived from what we eat. There are eight "essential" amino acids; these are not manufactured in the body as other amino acids are. Foods containing the eight "essential" amino acids are meats, fish, and eggs and are

TABLE 1. *Burning of calories for the average (154-pound) male*

		Activity burns it up if we			
Portion of food	Calories	Recline for	Walk for	Swim for	Run for
Butter, a pat	50	38 min	10 min	4.5 min	2.5 min
Large egg, one	80	61 min	15 min	7 min	4 min
Donut, one	125	1 hr 35 min	24 min	11 min	6 min
Beer, 12 oz.	150	1 hr 55 min	29 min	13 min	8 min

Source: *J. Amer. Diet Assoc.*, 46:186–188, 1965.

considered to be of high nutritional value. Beans, peas, and cereals contain protein of lesser value. Mixtures of the two types, however, make for tasty, less expensive meals.

Some animal food is necessary for a plentiful supply of protein. It is needed for growth, tissue repair, hemoglobin (the protein in the blood that carries oxygen from the lungs to tissues and then carries carbon dioxide from the tissues back to the lungs so it can be eliminated), and for disease-fighting antibodies.

Carbohydrates

Carbohydrates come as starches, sugars, and celluloses and fulfill our greatest energy needs. Cellulose, or plant fiber, has few calories but is necessary to normal bowel action. Adequate fiber or roughage in the diet is important to our lower bowel health.

Glucose, or blood sugar, is digested carbohydrates and, when absorbed into the blood, furnishes energy for body functions and growth. Carbohydrate saves protein for cell repair and helps in the breakdown of fat.

Starchy grains are eaten in pasta, bread, and cereal. Potatoes, sweet potatoes, dry beans, and peas and of course all the green vegetables also contain carbohydrates. Roughage or stool bulk is derived from whole grain cereals, vegetables, and fresh or dried fruit.

Fats

Fats are concentrated sources of energy and give twice the energy per gram of protein or carbohydrate. Fats take part in cell structure, cushion vital organs against trauma, and contain essential fatty acids.

Linoleic acid not produced from other fats in the body must be provided by our food, and it is found in many oils—corn, cotton seed, safflower, sesame seed, and soybean oil—and in wheat germ—all the polyunsaturated fats. Margarine and cooking oils come from these. Poultry fat and fish oils have more linoleic acid than do other sources.

It is best to keep the total amount of fat ingested moderate and to include sources of polyunsaturated fat. In addition to the oils above, fats are found in cream, cheese, nuts, chocolate, eggs, and meats.

Minerals and Vitamins

The best place to obtain minerals and vitamins is in the food you eat. Table 2 shows the mineral and vitamin content of 20 important foods.

Calcium is plentiful in the body. With phosphorus, it gives hardness to teeth and bones, where 99% of the body content of calcium resides. The small amount in other tissues and fluids ensures functioning of the heart, muscle, and nerves, and the coagulation of blood. Milk products are an excellent source, as are green vegetables and canned salmon (the kind with bones in).

Iodine prevents goiter and is found in seafood and in today's table salt.

Iron is needed in the formation of hemoglobin. Its content is very high in organ meats (liver, heart, and kidney), shellfish, egg yolk, green vegetables, and dried beans and peas.

Magnesium and *phosphorus* are important for bony structures and are found in whole grain products and dried peas and beans. If meals contain enough protein and calcium, phosphorus will automatically be contained in the diet. Another 10 minerals needed in trace amounts

TABLE 2. *Nutrient value of selected foods*

Nutrient	Unit	"Enriched" white bread	"Enriched" corn flakes	"Enriched" puffed rice	Cottage cheese
		I	I	I	II
Iodide	mg		(0.002–0.007)	(0.003)	
Cobalt	mg	0.0022	(0.0002)	(0.0006)	
Selenium	mg			0.002	
Molybdenum	mg	0.032	0.184		
Fluoride	mg				
Copper	mg	0.23	(0.06–0.08)	(0.06–0.19)	
Chromium	mg	0.003	0.004		
Manganese	mg	0.059	(0.15)	(1.08)	
Zinc	mg	0.97	(1.82)	(1.5)	
Iron	mg	2.5	1.4	1.8	0.4
Magnesium	mg	22.0	16.0	13–28	
Calcium	mg	84.0	17.0	20.0	90.0
Phosphorus	mg	97.0	45.0	92.0	175.0
Potassium	mg	105.0	120.0	100.0	72.0
Sodium	mg	507.0	1,005.0	2.0	290.0
Linoleic acid	g	Trace	(1)		Trace
Cholin	g		(0.06)		
Lysine	g	0.225	0.154	0.056	1.428
Methionine	g	0.142	0.135		0.469
Phenylalanine	g	0.465	0.354	0.286	1.099
Leucine	g	0.668	1.047		1.826
Valine	g	0.435	0.386		1.472
Isoleucine	g	0.429	0.306		0.989
Threonine	g	0.282	0.275		0.794
Tryptophan	g	0.091	0.052	0.046	0.179
Ascorbic acid (vitamin C)	mg	Trace	(0)	(0)	(0)
Niacin	mg	2.4	2.1	4.4	0.1
Vitamin E	mg	<0.23	(0.84)	(<0.23)	
Pantothenate	mg	0.43	0.185	0.378	0.22
Vitamin A	IU	Trace	(0)	(0)	10.0
Pyridoxine (vitamin B_6)	mg	0.04	0.065	0.075	0.04
Riboflavin (vitamin B_2)	mg	0.21	0.08	0.04	0.28
Thiamine (vitamin B_1)	mg	0.25	0.43	0.44	0.03
Folic acid	mg	0.015	0.0055	0.0076	0.0293
Vitamin K	mg				
Biotin	mg	0.0011	(0.0066)	0.0013	
Vitamin D	IU				
Cobalamine	μg	Trace	0	0	1.0
Miscellaneous					
Inositol	mg	51.0	(51)	19.0	
Cholesterol	mg				15.0
Fat	g	3.2	0.4	0.4	0.3
Protein	g	8.7	7.9	6.0	17.0
Carbohydrates	g	50.5	85.3	89.5	2.7
Water	% of	35.6	3.8	3.7	79.0
Calories	No.	270.0	386.0	399.0	86.0

Source: Williams, R. J. (1971): *Nutrition Against Disease.* Pitman, New York. This table, prepared by Dr. Roger J. Williams and his colleague Charles W. Bode at the University of Texas, Austin, is a more complete tabulation of nutrient contents than has appeared elsewhere.

TABLE 2. *(continued)*

American cheddar cheese	Whole milk (cow)	Fresh lettuce	Fresh tomatoes	Fresh oranges	Fresh carrots
II	II	III	III	III	III
	0.021	0.004	0.001–0.003		0.002
	0.006	0.005–0.023	0.009		
	0.02				
	0.016				
	0.019	0.04–0.15	0.06–0.11	0.07–0.31	0.34
	0.001				
	0.019	0.5–1.08	0.14	0.03	0.06–0.25
	0.35	0.18–0.47	0.24	0.17	0.11
1.0	Trace	2.0	0.5	0.4	0.7
45.0	13.0	11.0	14.0	11.0	23.0
750.0	118.0	35.0	13.0	41.0	37.0
478.0	93.0	26.0	27.0	20.0	36.0
82.0	144.0	264.0	244.0	200.0	341.0
700.0	50.0	9.0	3.0	1.0	47.0
1.0	Trace				
0.0453	0.015			0.012	0.013
1.834	0.272	0.07	0.042	0.024	0.052
0.65	0.086	0.004	0.007	0.003	0.01
1.34	0.17		0.016		0.042
2.437	0.344		0.014		0.065
1.794	0.24		0.022		0.056
1.685	0.223		0.029		0.046
0.929	0.161		0.033		0.043
0.341	0.049	0.012	0.009	0.003	0.01
(0)	1.0	8.0	23.0	50.0	8.0
0.1	0.1	0.3	0.7	0.4	0.6
1.0	0.1	0.29	0.27	0.23	0.45
0.5	0.34	0.2	0.33	0.25	0.28
1,310.0	140.0	970.0	900.0	200.0	11,000.0
0.08	0.04	0.055	0.1	0.06	0.15
0.46	0.17	0.06	0.04	0.04	0.05
0.03	0.03	0.06	0.06	0.1	0.06
0.015	0.0006	0.021	0.0037	0.00216	0.008
0.0033	0.0047	0.0031	0.004	0.00033	0.0025
1.0	0.40	0	0	0	0
23.3	13.0	51.0	46.0	120.0	48.0
100.0	11.0				
32.2	3.5	0.2	0.2	0.2	0.2
25.0	3.5	1.2	1.1	1.0	1.1
2.1	4.9	2.5	4.7	12.2	88.2
37.0	87.4	95.1	93.5	86.0	9.7
398.0	65.0	14.0	22.0	49.0	42.0

Dr. Williams emphasizes the incompleteness of our knowledge of the nutritive content of many common foods—and points up the uniqueness of each individual in his nutritional needs. There is an inability at this time on the part of medical science to tell us precisely what these requirements should be.

TABLE 2. *(continued)*

Nutrient	Unit	Raw potatoes	Whole chicken eggs	Medium quality beef	Pork
		III	IV	IV	IV
Iodide	mg		0.012		
Cobalt	mg	0.01	0.01	0.052	0.017
Selenium	mg	n.d.		0.028	<0.052
Molybdenum	mg	0.003	0.049	0.007	0.368
Fluoride	mg		0.06		
Copper	mg		0.17	0.09	0.39
Chromium	mg	0	0.016	0.009	0.01
Manganese	mg		0.04	0.005	0.034
Zinc	mg	0.868	1.3	5.66	1.89
Iron	mg	0.6	2.1	2.6	1.5
Magnesium	mg	22.0	9.0	21.0	20.9
Calcium	mg	7.0	54.0	10.0	6.0
Phosphorus	mg	53.0	210.0	155.0	103.0
Potassium	mg	407.0	149.0	300.0	285.0
Sodium	mg	3.0	111.0	65.0	70.0
Linoleic acid	g		2.2	Trace-1	5.0
Cholin	g	0.029	0.532	0.068	0.077
Lysine	g	0.107	0.87	1.45	0.804
Methionine	g	0.025	0.422	0.41	0.245
Phenylalanine	g	0.088	0.691	0.76	0.386
Leucine	g	0.1	1.09	1.35	0.721
Valine	g	0.107	1.05	1.0	0.51
Isoleucine	g	0.088	0.896	0.86	0.503
Threonine	g	0.079	0.704	0.735	0.455
Tryptophan	g	0.021	0.243	0.193	0.127
Ascorbic acid (vitamin C)	mg	20.0	0	0	(0)
Niacin	mg	1.5	0.1	4.2	2.7
Vitamin E	mg		2.0	0.47	0.63
Pantothenate	mg	0.4	2.7	0.47	0.5
Vitamin A	IU	Trace	1,140.0	45.0	(0)
Pyridoxine (vitamin B_6)	mg	0.22	0.25	0.33	0.46
Riboflavin (vitamin B_2)	mg	0.04	0.29	0.15	0.12
Thiamine (vitamin B_1)	mg	0.1	0.1	0.08	0.5
Folic acid	mg	0.0068	0.0094	0.009	0.0024
Vitamin K	mg				
Biotin	mg		0.0225	0.0026	0.0052
Vitamin D	IU				
Cobalamine	μg		0.282	1.42	
Miscellaneous					
Inositol	mg	29.0	33.0	11.5	45.0
Cholesterol	mg		550.0	70.0	70.0
Fat	g	0.1	12.8	23.0	52.0
Protein	g	2.1	11.5	23.0	10.2
Carbohydrates	g	17.1	0.7	0	0
Water	% of	79.8	74.0	54.0	37.3
Calories	No.	76.0	162.0	260.0	513.0

The figures given are for the quantities contained in 100 g of each food, approximately ¹/₄ pound. The second column indicates whether the quantity is grams

TABLE 2. *(continued)*

Lamb chops	Oysters	Peanuts	Beef liver	Brewer's yeast	Wheat germ
IV	IV	IV			
0.02	0.016	(0.026)	<0.016		0.0017
0.03	0.049	0.037	0.018		0.11
0.5	(0.01)	(0.1)	0.197		0.067
0.713	13.7	0.783	1.1	1.779	0.74
0.012	0.009	(0.035)			0.007
0.034	0.006	0.691	0.016		13.74
5.33	148.7	3.24	3.923	8.379	10.08
1.3	5.5	2.1	6.5	17.3	9.4
24.9	15.4	175.0	20.3	231.0	336.0
10.0	94.0	74.0	8.0	210.0	72.0
151.0	143.0	401.0	352.0	1,753.0	1,118.0
295.0	121.0	674.0	281.0	1,894.0	827.0
75.0	73.0	418.0	136.0	121.0	3.0
Trace		14.0	Trace		5.0
0.084		0.162	0.56	0.24	0.46
1.384		1.099	1.475	3.3	1.534
0.41		0.271	0.463	0.836	0.404
0.695		1.557	0.993	1.902	0.908
1.324		1.872	1.819	3.226	1.708
0.843		1.532	1.239	2.723	1.364
0.886		1.266	1.031	2.398	1.177
0.782		0.828	0.936	2.353	1.343
0.222		0.34	0.296	0.71	0.265
	30.0	0	31.0	Trace	(0)
4.9	2.5	17.2	13.6	37.9	4.2
0.62		4.6	1.4	0	12.5
0.59	0.49	2.13	7.7	12.0	3.3
	310.0		43,900.0	Trace	(0)
0.33	0.037	0.3	0.84	2.5	0.918
0.21	0.18	0.13	3.26	4.28	0.68
0.15	0.14	0.32	0.25	15.61	2.01
0.0033	0.0113	0.0566	0.293	2.2	0.305
0.0059	0.0087	0.034	0.1	0.2	(0.016)
			80.0	0	
58.0	44.0	180.0	51.0		770.0
70.0	>200.0		300.0		
22.6	1.8	49.3	3.8	1.0	10.9
16.8	8.4	26.0	19.9	38.8	26.6
0	3.4	18.8	5.3	38.4	46.7
59.3	84.6	1.6	69.7	5.0	11.5
276.0	66.0	585.0	140.0	283.0	363.0

(g), milligrams (mg), micrograms (μg), or international units (IU). (1g = 1,000 mg = 1,000,000 μg.)

will also be obtained if foods giving the minerals named above are eaten.

Vitamins play a dynamic role in body functions, in the release of energy from food, promoting normal growth, and ensuring proper functioning of all tissues. They are best obtained from foods.

Vitamin A is needed for normal growth and vitality, and it keeps the skin and inner linings of the body healthy. Outstanding sources of A are liver, eggs, whole milk, cheese, and the green and yellow vegetables.

Vitamin B—there are many B vitamins and they are called collectively the B-complex vitamins. They are all contained in Brewer's yeast. They release energy from food, help the nervous system to function, and are generously supplied in the meats we eat.

Vitamin D builds strong bones and teeth and functions in the body's utilization of calcium and phosphorus. Salmon, sardines, tuna, liver, and egg yolk are the best sources. Vitamin D is also produced in the skin under the influence of the sun and is absorbed in the general circulation.

Vitamin C, or ascorbic acid, keeps the body's form and maintains the cementing materials which hold body tissues together, strengthens the walls of blood vessels, and assists in healing processes.

The fact is that no diet for MS to date has been scientifically studied. There are no solid data to study, and we are faced with the unsupported claims of those who have advanced them. Usually claims are advanced with enthusiasm and at times with fanaticism. The claimants all protest, "If I can get the patient on my regimen early enough, my system will work." This statement of course ignores the fact that in the first years of MS there are several disappearances of symptoms, often complete ones—and occasionally symptoms never return.

Although a specific diet has not been studied, a dietary supplement has been. Seventy-five people with MS were studied in London and Belfast for 2 years using a linoleic acid source for the treated MS patients and an oleic acid source for the "control" MS subjects. Linoleic acid is an unsaturated fatty acid fat; oleic acid is a more saturated one. The investigators reported that the linoleic acid group had fewer acute attacks over the 2-year study, but the progress of the disease was the same in both groups.

Some dietary supplements, such as other unsaturated fatty acid fats, have been added to the diet in a controlled way, and these efforts too have led to disappointing results. Studies in England and Canada of linoleic acid preparations have failed to show differences in the groups studied.

Perhaps no scientist has come forward with a proposal for diet study in MS because such a study is difficult. It is difficult to plan and carry out. First, the diagnosis of MS in each patient must be confirmed by a special neurological team of doctors to be sure we have a study dealing with MS. For example, in groups referred by community physicians for diagnostic confirmation of MS by neurologists, 35% or more are rejected as not fulfilling the accepted international criteria for an MS diagnosis. Second, it is difficult to keep people on a given diet. Casual eating between meals is an almost unconscious act.

DIET AND URINARY INFECTION

Urinary incontinence may result from urinary tract infection (UTI), or from neurogenic bladder dysfunction, which predisposes the individual to bladder infections. Maintaining an acid urine—a medium unfavorable to the growth of causative organisms—helps prevent UTI. Dietary suggestions to help increase urinary acidity include the following:

1. Protein (meat, fowl, fish, eggs, and gelatin).
2. Large amounts of acidifying cranberries and their juice; plums and prunes. The cranberry juice provides a vitamin C substitute for citrus juices and is taken throughout the day, since excretion of vitamin C occurs rapidly. (Intake should be reduced at night to avoid nocturia and nocturnal enuresis.)

The following are foods that MS patients should try to eliminate from their diet when UTI is a problem: (1) Grapefruit, oranges, lemons, tomatoes, and their juices; (2) milk and its products; (3) beverages and antacids containing sodium carbonate or sodium bicarbonate (use Gelusil or other aluminum-type antacids instead); (4) noncitrus fruits and vegetables in large quantities, except those listed below; and (5) potatoes, lima beans, soy beans, greens, spinach, and dried vegetables.

As a substitute for potatoes, use two or more servings of white or brown rice, noodles, macaroni, spaghetti, or barley. Use cereals, preferably whole grain, dry or cooked; and sliced bread, preferably whole grain. For dessert: prune whips, gelatin, rice custard, bread pudding, tapioca, or custard pie. For nuts: filberts, walnuts, and Brazil nuts. Concentrated sweets may be taken. Fats that may be taken include butter, oil, nut butter, and cooking fats.

Elimination Problems

Constipation calls for the inclusion of bulk-producing bran combined with the daily use of one of the psyllium seed preparations; these absorb water and lead to moist stools. Water intake should be adequate. Prunes and prune juice also help reduce constipation.

These dietary measures need to be followed daily, since regulation of the digestive system is involved. If high-fiber intake, prunes, and adequate fluid ingestion do not successfully control constipation after a fair trial period, additional intervention procedures will need to be tried.

CONCLUSION

Adhering to a diet is a discipline, and discipline is a positive force within each of us. If the MS patient accepts this discipline, selects high-nutrient foods, and lives as full and independent and self-sufficient a life as possible, he or she can better deal with the challenges of living and coping with MS.

BIBLIOGRAPHY

The following are available from: Superintendent of Documents, U. S. Government Printing Office, Washington, D.C. 20402:

1. *Calories and Weight*, Agriculture Information Bulletin No. 364.

2. *Facts About Nutrition*, DHEW No. (NIH)74-423-1973, Stock No. 1740-00366.

3. *Food and Your Weight*, Agriculture Information Bulletin No. G 74.

4. *Food for Fitness*, Agriculture Information Bulletin No. L424.

5. *Nutritive Value of Foods*, Agriculture Information Bulletin No. G 72.

7

Physical and Surgical Therapy

Justin Alexander and Arthur S. Abramson

Questions are often asked about the effects of rest, activity, and exercise on MS. Does bed rest help or hinder recovery, especially during an acute attack? What level of activity should be maintained in the weakened or weakening individual? Are there specific benefits to be derived from exercise regimens? To the best of our knowledge, activity or rest has no effect on improving or worsening the disease process itself. However, they may have a definite effect on the more outward changes in the body that come about as a result of the disease. These are sometimes serious complications and can often be prevented by timely use of planned activity and rest. Such a regimen may also help to restore some degree of function and maintain it. The judicious use of various drugs, supportive devices, ambulatory aids, and certain surgical procedures are frequently of added benefit in this context.

There is a general principle that is operative in many individuals with progressive nervous system disorder. It is called "anticipation of disability." This means simply that those who are getting weaker tend to function below their actual capacity. As a matter of fact, it derives from a universal principle. None of us ever work up to our full capacity, a capacity determined by the fact that the human being possesses large untapped reserves of energy. If only half our potential were used normally, and if this tendency continued while our potential were being reduced by disease, we would be left with an insufficient display of energy to maintain an effective level of function. Thus the MS individual may discontinue extensive activity too early, may discontinue ambulation too early, and may even tend to become bed-bound too early. The problem is that underusing oneself may lead to the deleterious effects brought on by disuse. The nature of human tissue is such that it reacts to the kind of activity it is called on to perform. If such performance is inhibited, tissue and organs respond by reducing their substance and their function. For example, muscle shrinks (atrophy) and weakens if not used, bone loses its calcium and becomes fragile (osteoporosis), and underinflated lungs become easy prey to infection. This kind of process goes on in all tissues in which normal functioning is reduced or lost. Obviously, if inactivity tends to bring on such problems, activity should be effective in preventing, mitigating, or allaying them.

"Anticipation of disability" may be reinforced by another phenomenon that occurs in MS: the tendency to lassitude and fatigability. Individuals often report that they awaken refreshed in the morning and gradually feel more fatigued as the day passes, reaching a low point sometime in the late afternoon. There often is some recovery of vitality later in the evening. The probable reason for this characteristic cycle is that the fatigue appears to be related to the cycle of change in body temperature during the day. The core temperature of the body is usually lowest in the morning and at night and highest in the late afternoon. Of course, the difference between the lowest and highest points is not very great, and all levels usually are within what is considered the normal range unless the individual has a fever. Minor changes do not matter very much in the normal person, but nerve fibers of the individual with MS that have lost much of their waxy myelin coating in multiple parts of the nervous system are much more sensitive to very small rises in internal temperature. That this is so is shown by the rather remarkable increase in fatigue and the temporary worsening of the condition as determined by examination while being overheated by hot baths or by the environment on hot, humid days. In fact, in early cases where the diagnosis is still in doubt, the doctor may ask the patient to take a hot bath in order to raise the body temperature slightly, thereby causing physical signs to appear that are diagnostically helpful. Because of this phenomenon, individuals who are distressed by feeling fatigued are strongly advised to avoid hot baths and to keep as cool as they can on hot days even though the effects of overheating are only temporary.

Vigorous activity, especially exercising, also raises the internal temperature of the body slightly and may partially account for the rapid fatigue which occurs. For this reason it is advisable to intersperse short bouts of exercise with rest periods of at least equal duration to allow recovery to take place. This principle of exercise–rest–exercise–rest allows for the more effective use of restorative or fitness maintenance programs.

With the foregoing provisos in mind to prevent the abuses of rest, activity, and exercise, we can now discuss their uses. Physical functioning in the person with MS is hindered by weakness, stiffness (spasticity), and loss of coordination (ataxia). Not all necessarily occur at the same time or with the same degree of severity. Therefore each should be considered separately, even though at times they may tend to reinforce each other in terms of their deleterious effects on function.

WEAKNESS

Loss of strength and endurance is a prominent manifestation of MS. There are various ways in which such a loss can occur. It may be sudden, extensive, and severe (exacerbation), and it may last for days or even weeks after which the individual may gradually recover (remission). The recovery may not be complete, leaving some residual weakness. Several such episodes may occur, sometimes in rapid succession and sometimes with the lapse of years in-between. Alternatively, weakening may be a more gradual and continuing process without remissions. The speed of this process may vary considerably, from extreme rapidity to very slow progression. Fortunately, cases of very rapid progression are rare. On the other hand and more commonly, progression of the disability may be so slow that considerable function is retained for many years.

Cyclical and continuous types occasionally change from one to the other. In fact, there is a wide range of modes of weakening and no sure method of predicting their occurrence. In most instances, the weakness is usually not evenly distributed throughout the body. Both legs may be involved almost equally, or there may be a greater degree of involvement of just one leg. Less frequently, the same is true of the upper extremities. No matter what the type or location of the involvement, in the majority of people the ability to ambulate, even in the weakened state, may be retained for a very long time, especially with continued activity and exercise. The kind of activity and exercise that would be of therapeutic benefit is related to the type and location of the weakening process.

Exercise is most effective when used during recovery from an acute attack, that is, during the remitting stage. The pace and degree of recovery are increased by mobilizing latent potential by means of appropriate exercise. In this sense, the process is restorative. In the slowly and continuously progressive form of MS, exercise is designed to maintain rather than restore strength. In this way, "anticipation of disability" is not allowed to hold sway. In both of these examples, the residual state of the damaged nervous system ultimately dictates the optimal level of function possible as a result of restorative and maintenance programs.

During acute exacerbations and during the rapidly and continuously progressive form of the disease, exercise is much less effective although not harmful. In both cases, the progression of the disability may be more rapid than any benefits to be expected from physical therapy. As a matter of fact, some doctors recommend bed rest rather than activity. It must be remembered, however, that total inactivity promotes the appearance of the maximal deleterious metabolic effects of the process of disuse. For example, it is during prolonged periods of bed rest that pressure sores over bony prominences (decubitus ulcers) tend to form because of the poor nutritional status of tissues which normally resist pressure. Unless there is meticulous attention paid to nursing care of the bedridden patient, including frequent turning of the individual with close inspection of the skin over pressure areas, these ulcers are a danger.

If any large group of people with MS were asked the function they would prefer to maintain, the majority would probably choose the ability to walk effectively. There are a number of disorders which place effective walking in jeopardy (such as weakness, spasticity, and loss of coordination). Activities, especially walking, depend on strength, endurance, speed, and coordination.

In order to increase strength, the muscle groups which perform movements must be worked against the heaviest loads they can carry. This must be done against gravity and through the full range of movements. Special attention must be paid to the antigravity muscles, such as those of the calves, front of the thighs, the rear muscles which straighten the hips, and the muscles of the lower back. It is the weakening of these muscles which makes walking in the erect position so difficult. Because the resistance afforded by externally applied loads is maximal, only a very few repetitions through complete range of motion can be tolerated. However, even these few repetitions, repeated daily, may be sufficient, providing the damage to the nervous system is not enough to deny improvement of strength. Heavy resistance exercise is quite a popular form of physical therapy and is sometimes done with fans blowing air over exercising MS patients to keep them cool. It must be remembered that the maximal load tolerated depends on the degree of residual strength, being greater in the stronger person and less in the weaker.

Training for endurance must be done differently. Endurance cannot be built up with only a few repetitions of the movements, as training for strength alone does not necessarily provide endurance. Many repetitions are required during exercise to fulfill the need for prolonged activity not requiring great strength, which is the usual situation in daily living. Therefore the load during these exercises is only a fraction of that required when building up strength. The smaller the load, the more repetitions are possible. Ideally, loads should be chosen which compare to those encountered in the activities of daily living.

It should be obvious from the foregoing that some professional help is needed when the patient is learning how to exercise for building strength and endurance. Therefore the physician will usually prescribe a few sessions with a skilled physical therapist, who will teach patients how to do these exercises by themselves and in their own homes. They are, of course, designed for individuals who are still strong enough to walk, even though poorly. Such vigorous exercises are often beyond the capacity of the individual who is too weak to walk. The exercises can only improve pre-existing movements, not create them.

SPASTICITY

Damage to the central nervous system usually causes some degree of spasticity. Spasticity is due to involuntary muscle contractions, and the relaxation from these contractions is also involuntary. Spasticity is stimulated by changes in posture, mainly by stretching some muscles and contracting others. This is exactly what happens when the MS patient is walking: The weakened muscles still under voluntary control tend to act in an orderly pattern, some contracting while others relax. While doing so they coincidentally stimulate a pattern of involuntary (spastic) contractions, not an orderly process. Muscles contract excessively here, including those that are supposed to be relaxing. As a result, the individual's gait becomes labored, stiff, and slow because voluntary movement is now fighting involuntary movement.

The added muscle action of spasticity may enable an individual to stand even though voluntary control may be not quite enough to do so by itself. However, because more muscle mass is being used than is necessary for graceful walking, the energy costs are so increased that endurance is markedly reduced. The individual who has sufficient voluntary control, and who would be able to walk more easily, farther, and better without spasticity, will reach an early point of exhaustion with it. In addition, spasticity tends to stiffen knees and hips, and push down the feet. The ability to step high enough to clear the feet from the walking surface is lost. This becomes an especially difficult problem when mounting stairs and going uphill. It is also not compatible with skilled use of the arms and hands when, less frequently, the upper extremities become involved in the spasticity process.

Spasticity has become increasingly manageable in recent years thanks to the introduction of reasonably effective antispasticity drugs.

Although these agents eliminate all stiffness, by titrating the dosage they may reduce spasticity enough that the individual can function more effectively using less energy. There are a number of drugs that can produce this result, but some have other, less desirable effects as well. They may weaken voluntary motion or excessively tranquilize the individual when given in doses that reduce the spasticity.

Fortunately, there are drugs which concentrate mostly on the spasticity. Such drugs are begun in very small doses and then are increased every 3 or 4 days until the best possible effect is obtained. The top dose varies from one individual to another and depends on the severity of the spasticity. When the underlying weakness and the spasticity are both severe, there is a point, when adjusting the dosage, that the legs may become rubbery because support of the spasticity is diminished. The patient's ability to stand and even his labored walking are now jeopardized. This is a signal to revert to the next lower dose. Even the minimal effect of a small dose is valuable as the individual will quickly discover if the antispasticity drug is completely withdrawn.

A destabilizing effect of the drugs in the individual who is not ambulatory, who has good upper extremities, but who also has very severe and uncomfortable spasticity in the legs is not a major concern. Therefore large doses can be used in this patient so that he is more comfortable sitting in a wheelchair or lying in bed. The individual with strong underlying voluntary motion whose gait is awkward and exhausting because of excessive spasticity should also be given larger doses as they would not threaten his ability to walk.

With appropriate use of antispasticity medication, walking may be improved still further by supporting the dropped feet. Laminated polyethylene short leg braces are usually prescribed for this purpose. They fit within the shoes and are not unsightly. They keep the toes clear of the ground, further reducing the energy needed to walk.

When weakness and spasticity become excessive, the ability to function is markedly reduced, and the individual tends to be relegated to the wheelchair or may even begin spending much of the day in bed. This creates a vicious cycle because the effects of disuse created by these circumstances reduce function still further. Activity can be maintained in this situation by using underwater activity as therapy. The buoyancy of lukewarm water in a swimming pool eliminates much of the disabling forces of gravity and allows for a degree of function no longer possible on dry land (such as walking). Water also provides some resistance to movement, which is beneficial in enhancing strength. Regular sessions in the swimming pool should be part of the regimen to maintain fitness.

Spasticity, especially when unevenly distributed, may tend to produce deformities that can develop as further barriers to effective walking. In the commonest example, the inner thigh muscles sometimes become so excessively hyperactive that gait will take on a scissoring appearance. If the hyperactivity is greater on one side, that leg will be pulled inward, pushing up the pelvis on that side in an attempt to keep the leg in a straight up-and-down posture. This tilting of the pelvis will also curve the spine away from the midline and perhaps throw it off balance. Because of the tilt up, the leg seems to be shorter. When such deformities are sustained over a long time, the muscles gradually adapt their lengths to the distorted postures and the deformities become more difficult to correct. This deforming propensity of spasticity may occur in other areas as well.

The tendency to deformation must be combated by applying counterbalancing forces regularly. Such forces are supplied by what is known as "passive stretching" exercises. Joints are carried through their full range of motion periodically making sure that muscles are stretched to their full lengths. This will mitigate against deforming postures being long sustained and prevent them from becoming fixed. The exercises should be done on a daily basis and often require the help of a family member. They are easier to perform when antispasticity drugs are used to lessen the resistance of muscles to stretching.

Occasionally a spastic contraction is so strong that the response to these exercises is less than hoped for. When that occurs, "nerve blocks" may be tried. Injecting an anesthetic around the nerve that leads to the the hip weakens those muscles sufficiently that immediately after the block the individual may be able to walk without scissoring and even use less energy. If this proves to be effective in a particular individual, a longer-lasting nerve block with a solution of phenol can maintain the weakening effect for 6 months or longer; it sometimes even has a permanent effect. If the anesthetic does not provide relief, its effect will pass off quickly with no harm done, and another form of management will have to be considered.

Although the inner thigh muscles are useful in walking, they are not absolutely essential. People have been known to walk well with these muscles completely paralyzed. Other excessively contracting muscle groups that can produce deformity may be more important for walking. Fortunately, the technique of temporary nerve blocking can determine very quickly whether walking is possible, and it is a rather simple and not a frightening procedure.

When the deformity is fixed and not reversible through blocking, more radical procedures are called for, such as cutting the tendons of offending muscles. The tendons will rejoin over time but will be of greater length, making the muscles attached to them that much shorter and therefore weaker. This, in a sense, produces a result similar to that of nerve blocking in patients without fixed deformity. The main drawback to cutting tendons is that an overcorrected position must be maintained for several weeks by splints of a plaster cast so that the gap between the cut ends of the tendon will be filled in by the longest possible new tendon. An intensive course of physical therapy immediately following removal of the splints or cast should rapidly reverse the effects of the weeks of inactivity and should rapidly gain and retain a new and improved pattern of gait.

LOSS OF COORDINATION

Loss of coordination could be a most difficult problem for the person with MS. Fortunately, it does not always occur. When it does, it often does not progress to the point of overwhelming disability, and sometimes it undergoes spontaneous remission. There are no truly effective drugs to control it, and exercise therapy is usually of minimal benefit except perhaps if the loss is mild. Loss of coordination manifests in several ways. Every individual with MS should be familiar with the finger-to-nose and heel-to-shin tests which are performed during the physical examination. The more the arm or leg wavers in performing these tests (intention tremor) the greater the loss of coordination of the upper or lower extremities. When the wavering is only slight, the legs and arms still have their usefulness. This symptom is not always evenly distributed. It can be mild or almost nonexistent in the extremities yet become evident on walking. In that case, the gait would be unstable, with a tendency to stagger to one side or the other, especially on turning; this occasionally leads to a fall.

Above all, gait must be kept within safe limits, and for this purpose walking aids should be used to stabilize locomotion. These aids can afford different degrees of stability depending on how broad a supporting base is being offered. If only slight stabilization is needed, a simple cane would be enough, and it is usually used on the side toward which the individual staggers. A cane with four supporting points at the base (quad cane) broadens the supporting surface still further and is indicated when greater stabilization is needed. The proper height of a cane is determined by standing upright with the cane held at the side. The height is correct when the elbow is at a 30 degree angle in this position.

Finally, the broadest base affording the greatest degree of stability is provided by a walker. This is a light aluminum structure with two supporting points on either side. Its proper height is determined as it is for a cane. The walker is lifted and advanced prior to each step. The type that can be folded, making it easy to transport, is preferable.

We recently saw a patient who had not walked for 9 years because of an unstable gait. Examination revealed adequate strength and only minimal spasticity and loss of coordination of the arms and legs. There was no evidence that the disease had worsened over these years. Unfortunately, no one had thought of providing her with walking aids. Upon being presented with a walker, she was able to walk safely and for considerable distances with minimal training. This is a glaring example of lost opportunity because of neglect in using walking aids. Fortunately it does not occur often.

There are some who resist the use of aids because they do not like the appearance. They pay the price of staying home with restricted movement because of lack of safety or because they might appear to be intoxicated to others in public. There is no shame in helping oneself, especially if one profits by it with increased activity and widened horizons.

A trial of therapeutic exercise should be considered in all forms of disability including loss of coordination. However, it should not be continued endlessly if there are no favorable results—and such results should become apparent within a few weeks. If gains do occur, however, they cannot be expected to continue forever because that is saying that exercise can restore normality and, in most cases, that is not possible. When gains are achieved they should be maintained by self-activation. The best exercise is to use oneself maximally and thus prevent "anticipation of disability." The type of exercise that can be used by the individual with mild to moderate loss of coordination is described later.

NONAMBULANT INDIVIDUAL

To this point we have considered the individual who is still walking to some extent. However, the progression of the disease may reach a point when walking is no longer possible despite every effort to restore and maintain it. Prior to this time and when ambulation has become extremely taxing, the use of a wheelchair for longer distance is called for. This makes the transition to total nonambulation easier and maintains the range of the individual's activities. For those with useful arm motion, wheelchairs can maintain fitness because of the energy demanded to move the chair. If that becomes too exhausting or if the upper extremities are too weak or uncoordinated to move the chair effectively, various types of battery-powered chairs and vehicles are available. Selection of an appropriate wheelchair requires an evaluation of the person's ability to move, to transfer, the environment in which the person will be using the chair, and a knowledge of what is available. A physical therapist can provide assistance in picking the best chair for any person.

When walking is no longer possible, the ability to propel a wheelchair is not enough. The person must be able to transfer from bed to wheelchair, from wheelchair to another seat (as in theaters, autos, or toilets), and into a shower or bath. To accomplish this, transfer training may be required. The principles underlying such training are simple. They consist of: (a) strengthening the muscles of the arms and shoulders so that they can lift the trunk and carry it for short distances; (b) learning what supporting surfaces can be used most effectively in making transfers; and (c) how to use sliding boards when arms are weak. Often transfer maneuvers can be done by the patient himself, although occasionally some assistance is required. If the patient has maintained a range of locomotion and the ability to transfer himself, work and avocational and recreational pursuits should be restricted only minimally.

OTHER EXERCISE REGIMENS

No discussion of the uses of exercise would be complete without mentioning certain special types which have their enthusiastic advocates. Chief among them are facilitation and biofeedback exercises. Facilitation exercises comprise a number of systems most often labeled with the names of the originators of the systems. They are quite complex and require experienced therapists for their application.

Despite their apparent variety, a common principle governs all of them. When the central nervous system has been damaged, it tends to become overly excitable. That is the basis for the development of spasticity. The hyperexcitable nervous system responds to many kinds of stimulation which in normal circumstances it would not do. The response consists largely of muscle contraction.

The facilitation exercise systems are based on the fact that certain muscles which enhance desired movements respond to the right kind of stimuli at the right places. Stimuli are supplied by changes in the posture of specific parts of the body or by brushing or tapping certain skin areas. There is a doctrine developed around the relationship between the kinds of stimuli, the place to be stimulated, and the specific muscles which will respond.

Unfortunately, there is no clear-cut evidence that increased strength, endurance, and range of voluntary movement result from the facilitation exercises. Nevertheless, practitioners of these methods often claim good results. For this reason, they may be worth a therapeutic trial during a stable period (remission). Proponents of this technique suggest that "plasticity" of the nervous system permits motion elicited through enforcement to eventually become voluntary and thereby functional.

Biofeedback training is of more recent vintage. It is based on the amplification of electrical signals produced by muscle contraction so that the individual can see the result of even minimal voluntary contraction on a television-like screen or hear the signals from a loudspeaker. Seeing and hearing small contractions, even those that are insufficient to produce any meaningful movement, is a motivating force in attempting to increase the size and volume of what is being seen and heard, and so perhaps to achieve increased movement. It is really a refinement of exercise therapy where more visible small movements motivate the individual to strive for larger ones. It is also used in an attempt to inhibit excessive muscle activity as in spasticity. Unfortunately, its role in treatment is not yet clearly established. After all, it is meant to enhance existing voluntary motion, not to create it. It does not have the magical ability to translate involuntary to voluntary motion. Ultimately, the remaining intact part of the nervous system will determine what is possible, and that can be done in most cases by more traditional forms of physical therapy.

In summary, there is a role for exercise therapy in restoring or maintaining function. The extent to which this is possible is limited by the nature and degree of damage to the nervous system, by the severity of weakness, spasticity, and incoordination, and by fatigability. The tendency to anticipate disability that leads to the constitutional effects of disuse is reversible. Exercise therapy is designed to increase strength, endurance, speed, and coordination. The use of certain drugs, nerve blocks, supporting devices, walking aids, and occasionally surgery may be of help in this process. The major role of self-help and self-activation is emphasized. To this end, a personal exercise regimen is outlined.

PERSONAL EXERCISE REGIMEN

Length of muscles can be maintained by ensuring that all joints of limbs are moved through their complete range at least once daily. It may, however, require more than one attempt to gain this objective. The exercises can be done independently or, if necessary, with the aid of other persons. The exercises described here are only some that can be performed. Generally they should be done on one side and then repeated on the other unless specifically designated as bilateral (or symmetrical). For best results they should be discussed with a physical therapist to ensure that they are performed correctly.

Facelying—Preferably on a Firm Surface

1. *Lift the leg off the floor about 5 inches with knee straight, hold, and return to starting position.*
If help is required, the assistant should cradle the leg in one arm and press with the other hand on the patient's buttock to ensure that the motion occurs at the hip joint. If the goal of exercising is to strengthen the muscles, resistance should be applied. This can take the form of pressure exerted by the "helper" on the buttock (for stabilization) and over the back of the knee joint. Resistance should not be so heavy as to prevent motion, but enough to constitute a challenge.

Resistance can also be applied by means of a sand bag, a bag filled with canned goods, or other easily available objects. An exercise boot with plate weights can be obtained from any store that sells sporting goods. "Cuff weights" are very easy to use for almost any body part. Some have provisions for varying the weight.

2. *Keeping the hip and buttocks fixed, bend the knee back.*
Normal range is about 110 to 120 degrees from the fully straightened position. If assistance is required, stabilization should be provided

over the hip and back of the thigh, cradling the lower leg. This ensures better control of motion. Manual resistance can be applied over the back of the ankle, and a pulley with weights can also be employed to provide resistance.

3. *Keeping the hip and knee fixed, push the foot down as far as possible, as if attempting to stand on the toes.*
Resistance can be applied against this motion by leaning the assistant's thigh against the sole of the foot. However, easier alternatives to this technique are described.

4. *Holding on to a fixed point with the arms extended over the head, attempt to lift both legs 3 to 5 inches off the supporting surface.*
This is an excellent exercise to strengthen low back muscles.

5. *With arms resting along the body, lift both arms about 10 inches off the surface.*
Some find it helpful to hold on to a stick. This is especially recommended when one arm is weaker. If assistance is required, one arm at a time is exercised. Stabilization should be applied over the shoulder, and the arm should be cradled. Manual resistance can be applied over the elbow, and of course the patient can hold any type of weight in the hand.

6. *With hands clasped behind the low back, squeeze shoulders together and attempt to lift the head and shoulders from the surface.*
Exercise can be made more challenging by clasping the hands behind the head and finally by holding a weight in that fashion.

7. *Push-ups—place both hands on the floor at the level of the shoulder and slowly straighten both elbows, thereby raising head, chest, and as much of the trunk as possible from the floor. Hold to a count of five and slowly lower the body back to the floor.*
A modified push-up requires only the raising of head and upper trunk.

Hands and Knees Position

1. *Lower the head and simultaneously round the back by tightening stomach muscles. Then raise the head and allow the back to sag down, giving a swayback appearance.*

2. *Balance exercise*

a. *Head up—shift weight to right, divide weight-bearing on all fours; shift weight to the left.*

b. *Head up—shift weight to right and raise left arm, lower arm, shift weight to all fours, shift weight to left, raise right arm.*

c. *Head up—lift left arm and right leg, relax, lift right arm and left leg.*

d. *Raise trunk to kneeling poisition, lift arms to side or forward.*

Assistant may gently push against the trunk to increase balance response.

Backlying

1. *Straight leg raising—with arms at the side, lift each leg as high as possible, keeping the knee straight and pelvis flat against the floor.*

If assistance is required, stabilization occurs over the pelvis and the leg should be cradled. If the posterior thigh muscles (hamstrings) are tight and need to be stretched, the assistant should kneel in front of the patient, place the patient's leg on his (the assistant's) shoulder, clasp hands over the patient's knee and *slowly* straighten up while maintaining pressure over the knee.

This same exercise can be modified to increase the strength of the hip flexors by stabilizing over the pelvis and offering manual resistance over the knee. Weights can be used quite easily for this purpose.

2. *Spread the legs apart, symmetrically when possible.*

A variation of this exercise involves hooking one leg over the edge of the bed or any other fixed point and moving the other leg.

If assistance is required, the helper can move one leg at a time, cradling the moving leg and holding the other one; or he can grasp both heels and then move the legs apart. Some people find it easier to kneel between the patient's legs and push with their own legs to stretch the adductors.

Spreading the legs can be used for several purposes. If inner thigh muscles (adductors) are tight, stretching can be achieved in this manner. Resistance to spreading the legs can be used to increase muscle strength necessary to maintain a level pelvis, thus enabling standing, or to move the leg out to the side (abductors). When both legs are moved simultaneously, resistance is given on the outer aspect of the ankle. If one leg is moved at a time, stabilization of the pelvis with one hand is essential. Resistance can be applied at the outer aspect of the knee.

3. *Sit-ups* can be used to strengthen abdominal muscles. Knees should be bent and held firmly by the assistant. If no assistant is available, the feet can be hooked under a firm support (low couch). Exercise should initially be performed with the arms straight out in front, lifting the head and shoulders up. It is important that the head is kept well forward at all times. The exercise can be progressed by folding the arms over the chest and finally behind the back of the head.

4. *Place the right hand on the left shoulder, extending the left arm. As the body is raised the left arm reaches toward the right hip and knee. Repeat to the opposite side: with left hand on right shoulder and right arm extended, sit up and reach toward left hip and knee.*

This is a modification of the sit-up that can be performed to include trunk rotator muscles.

5. *Sit with knees straight and reach toward the toes.*

This stretches the back extensor muscles. Assistance can be provided by the helper kneeling behind the patient and gently pushing the head and upper trunk forward. If knees are kept fixed, the hamstrings will also be stretched.

6. *Move to the edge of a raised surface until one leg can be bent at the knee over the edge of the table; the other leg is then raised until the foot can rest on the surface. Straighten the leg hanging over the edge of the table.*

Resistance can be applied by a weighted boot, cuff weight, pulleys with weight, or an assistant. In the latter case the helper pushes against the leg just in front of the ankle. It is also recommended that the other arm be placed under the leg being exercised and the foot of the resting leg held by that hand. When using mechanical resistance, a small towel roll under the knee being exercised is quite helpful.

7. *Bend toes and ankle toward the head as if standing on the heel.*

This stretches the heel cord and can be used to increase the strength of the muscles that allow ambulation without stubbing one's big toes (dorsiflexors). Resistance can be supplied by the assistant's hand over the top of the foot, by sand bags, or by cuff weights.

8. *Hold onto a stick with both hands, and let arms lay straight along the body. Raise both arms as high as possible above the head, keeping the elbows straight.*

An assistant can help to continue the motion if muscle tightness prevents reaching the target. To use this exercise for strengthening, plate weights, sand bags, or cuff weights can be attached to the stick.

9. *Hold onto a stick and, with elbows bent and hands next to the shoulders, push up to the ceiling.*

Resistance can be added as described above.

Sitting in a Wheelchair

One of the most important exercises to be performed in the wheelchair provides a means of strengthening elbow extensors (triceps) and at the same time is an effective technique for preventing pressure sores on the buttocks.

1. *Place hands on the armrests of the chair and straighten the elbows. Hold to the count of three and slowly lower the body back into the seat.*

The whole body can be raised from the chair in this fashion. Guard against allowing the shoulders to be elevated. If the legs cannot be raised concomitantly with the rest of the body, just raising the buttocks off the seat will do. This exercise should be performed at least 5 to 10 times every hour while sitting up.

2. *Arms in lap, raise arms as high as possible and breathe in deeply. Let arms down and exhale.*

3. *With the arms straight toward the floor, bend the arm, bringing the hand toward the shoulder.*

Resistance can be offered by means of various weights and pulleys, or by an assistant who places one hand just proximal to the elbow, holding the upper arm steady and giving resistance over the wrist.

4. *Lean forward and reach toward the floor. Then raise trunk, shoulders, and head. Do not use your arms; try to start straightening at the low back.*
Breathing exercises can be combined with this exercise.

5. *Raise one knee at a time toward the chest. Keep the trunk steady. Hold to a count of three and let the leg down. Repeat with other leg.*
Resistance can be given by means of a weighted boot, sand bag, or cuff weights. An assistant can apply pressure over the thigh just above the knee.

6. *Straighten the knee until the lower leg and thigh are in a straight line. If muscle tightness interferes with this motion, rest one leg on a chair (with a cushion under the heel to prevent skin breakdown) and place a weight over the knee. Allow the muscle to stretch for about 15 to 20 minutes. It is important to sit straight.*
If resistance is needed, a weighted boot, sand bag, or cuff weights can be used. An assistant places one arm under the exercising knee, resting a hand on the stationary knee, and provides resistance by pushing against the lower leg just above the ankle.

7. *Place the heel of one leg over the ankle of the other. Slide heel to the knee and down. Watch the leg closely while performing the exercise. Try the same exercise with eyes closed.*
Modify the above exercise by raising the heel from the other leg and placing it at preselected points of the leg. The assistant can touch the point to which the heel is to be raised. First use visual guidance, then attempt it without watching.

Standing

1. *While holding on to a stable support (avoid coffee tables, etc.), stand on one leg and then raise up to the toes. Repeat until the exercise can be performed 10 times.*

2. *Place a series of adhesive tape strings on the floor about 12 to 18 inches apart in a staggered fashion to provide a guide for*

placing the feet when walking. Attempt to walk touching each piece of tape with the leading foot.

3. Dance to slow music.

This is an excellent way of improving balance.

Selection of specific exercises should be based on the particular need of an individual. It is best to select a limited number of the most important exercises to be done at one time. Exercising must be built into the daily schedule as much as any other normal activity. The program should be reviewed periodically by the physical therapist to ensure that it is still correct and to permit modifications.

8

Aids to Ease the Activities of Daily Living

Kate Robbins and Arthur S. Abramson

MS often results in difficulty walking and in using the arms and hands because of weakness, spasticity, and loss of coordination. Visual and sensory difficulties may also occur. These do not necessarily occur together, nor are they all inevitable. They may occur rather suddenly, last for a while, and then improve; or they may occur slowly with less likelihood of improvement. In either case there may be a reduction in the ability to walk effectively or to adequately perform the activities we encounter in daily living.

This chapter is intended as a guide for finding the safest ways to keep functioning by using satisfactory rehabilitation equipment and environmental and or architectural modifications when necessary. It is directed to the MS patient him- or herself.

MOBILITY

If you have problems walking, you have probably already arranged your environment to make it easier for you to get around. This may mean having heavy pieces of furniture in your home or work space placed along common pathways to provide support, or grab bars may have been installed for a secure handhold. Often this manner of "furniture walking" is adequate only in a space you know well and have arranged to suit your needs; elsewhere some sort of walking aid—cane, forearm crutch, or walker—may greatly increase your stability and therefore your mobility. To determine which aid will offer you the greatest stability and safety requires discussion with your physician or physical therapist, who can instruct you in the best way for you to walk with the aid, go through doorways, sit down and get up from a chair, enter and leave a car, etc. This will vary somewhat depending on which walking aid you use, how you use it, and what works best (most safely) for you.

Maintaining mobility and reducing energy expenditure will be enhanced by one common-sense rule: Sit when conditions permit. Your energy is thus saved for mobility when that becomes necessary. For instance, place chairs in major work areas in your kitchen or office, or bring all the work to one area (perhaps on a wheeled utility cart); arrange major supermarket shopping by phone or go during off hours when there are not long checkout lines. Only a general rule is offered here; you should decide how best to work it into your life style.

WHEELCHAIRS AND MOBILITY

If you are easily tired by walking, you may choose to use a wheelchair (W/C) some of the time to conserve energy and to enhance your range of locomotion, or you may use a W/C if your legs are very weak. Folding W/Cs are preferred because they can be placed in a car for travel and folded out of the way when not in use. Choosing the best W/C to serve you should be discussed with a rehabilitation specialist: an occupational therapist, physical therapist, or physiatrist.

Guidelines used in choosing the most appropriate W/C are a person's size, the easiest means of maneuvering the chair (manually or by motor), and the specific environment in which it will be used. The two most common W/C sizes are the standard adult W/C (seat measures 18 inches in width and 16 inches in depth, backrest extends 16.5 inches above the seat, overall width is 24.5 to 26 inches) and the narrow adult W/C (seat measures 16 inches in width and depth, backrest extends 16.5 inches above the seat, overall width is 22.5 to 24.5 inches). Slim adult W/Cs (seat width is only 14 inches) and wide adult W/Cs (seat widths up to 24 inches) are also available. A short adult may be most comfortable in a junior, or low seat, model that is closer to the ground. The tall adult W/C has a 1-inch greater seat depth (17 inches) and a 1.5-inch greater seat height (18 inches), with the standard adult seat width of 18 inches or the narrow adult seat width of 16 inches. An exceptionally tall, large, or small person may want to special order a W/C from a manufacturer.

When seated, your thighs should be parallel to the W/C seat (knees should not be tilted upward), with a 2- to 3-inch space between the edge of the seat and the back of your knees. The W/C seat should extend no more than 1 inch on either side of you and should provide firm support. If the seat begins to sag, replace the upholstery or use a solid seat insert, which is a solid board and a layer of foam rubber covered by vinyl. The solid seat insert should be placed between the seat rails, not on them. Some manufacturers can provide a solid folding seat which allows the solid seat to remain attached to the W/C even when it is folded.

The backrest should be high enough to provide adequate support but not interfere with shoulder movement. A backrest that is wider (flared) at the top or a headrest can provide more upper body support. If weakness and/or spasticity make it difficult for you to sit upright in a wheelchair, a semireclining back and a wedge-shaped seat cushion will tilt you back slightly (10 to 30 degrees) to prevent your "sliding out." A semireclining back increases the overall length of a W/C by 3 inches.

Armrests may be stationary (part of the W/C frame) or removable (slipped into and out of tubular supports). Whether stationary armrests or removable armrests are chosen depends on how you transfer from the W/C. If you stand up to transfer, stationary armrests are fine; but if you sometimes slide out of the W/C sideways with a sliding board, you will need removable armrests. (When purchasing a W/C, remember that stationary and removable armrests are not interchangeable. If you purchase a W/C with stationary armrests and later need removable armrests, you will have to purchase a new W/C.) The armrest should be at a comfortable height, so that your elbows and forearms rest naturally on them. If the armrests are too low, your shoulders will droop. If the armrests are too high, your shoulders will be pushed upward. Either position soon becomes uncomfortable. Correct armrest height can be achieved by raising your height in the W/C with a cushion, a combination of a solid seat and a cushion, or if the armrests are removable by choosing height-adjustable armrests that can be adjusted from 8¾ to 13¾ inches above the seat. W/C desk arms have a shorter armrest and therefore permit a closer approach by the W/C to desks and tables. Removable desk arms can be inserted into the wheelchair with the higher part of the rests toward the back for closer approaches to furniture, or toward the front for easier standing transfers. Removable armrests increase the overall width of a W/C by 1.5 inches. Wrap-around removable armrests do not increase the width because they slip into supports behind the backrest. If you need to use removable armrests, the reduction in W/C width makes wrap-around armrests a wise choice. It is obvious that the narrower the chair the more doors you will be able to go through because doors come in many widths.

Swinging detachable footrests with standard or large footplates are usually recommended. They can be adjusted to your leg length and can swing out of the way or detach completely from the W/C for a closer approach to bed, toilet, bathtub, etc. Heel loops on the footplates or a strap or panel behind your legs may be helpful if your feet slip off the footplates. Swinging detachable elevating legrests elevate as well as swing out of the way and detach. Your doctor may recommend them if your legs tend to swell because of being in the down position too long, or you may prefer them for comfort. Elevating legrests are somewhat heavier when you push the chair or detach and reattach them.

Hard rubber tires (the large back wheels) and casters (the small front wheels) are the narrowest available (1¼ inches) and are easiest to push across smooth indoor surfaces. Semipneumatic and pneumatic tires and casters are wider (1¾ to 2 inches) and better for maneuvering across thick carpets or soft bumpy ground. If you have difficulty grasping the hand rims to propel the W/C, they may be fitted with rubber covers to improve your grip, or projections or knobs may be attached to the hand rim. Wider tires and hand rim projections increase the overall width of the W/C.

The variety of W/C accessories is considerable, including plastic shields to protect fingers from spinning spokes, long-handled brake extensions, cane/crutch holders, lap boards, carrying pouches, cup holders, and ashtrays. A narrowmatic or reduce-a-width attachment can temporarily reduce the width of a folding W/C as much as 4 inches. By turning a handle *while the W/C is moving*, you actually cause the chair to start folding up. This will not work with any solid seat and should be used only while passing through a narrow doorway or hallway. Even W/C carrying racks that can be attached to the back of a small car are available. Your dealer or manufacturer can provide you with a complete list of accessories and related items. It is of no use to load a W/C with every accessory, only those for which there is an evident need.

A seat or backrest cushion is not considered an accessory. New cushion material and designs are continually being developed by manufacturers and tested at rehabilitation centers, so there may be more than one type of cushion that is adequate for your needs. (That spare throw pillow you have lying around the house is *not* adequate.) According to your weight and body structure, a rehabilitation specialist will be able to help you choose the proper cushion or combination of cushions for good posture and stability, prevention of skin breakdown, ease in transfers, and comfort. Avoid extremely heavy cushions; these are difficult to lift out of the W/C and may provide less protection against skin breakdown. Vinyl covers that protect cushions from moisture may also be uncomfortable to sit on, especially in warm weather. A thick terry towel wrapped around the vinyl, or sewn to fit over the vinyl cover, will make the cushion more comfortable and is easily washed.

Motorized W/Cs, with the motor and batteries mounted underneath, are similar in appearance to manual wheelchairs. Some manual wheelchairs can even be converted to the motorized variety. Control boxes are placed near the right or left armrest for hand control. Adaptations for chin or breath (sip 'n puff) control can also be made for the very few extremely disabled. Before purchasing a motorized W/C, it is best to evaluate your ability with the various controls at a rehabilitation center. Motorized W/Cs are very expensive; and though after removing the batteries some can be folded for car or plane travel, they are much heavier than manual W/Cs and require meticulous maintenance.

An increasingly popular alternative to motorized W/Cs are the less-expensive motorized scooters. A scooter operator should have good sitting stability and be able to reach forward with at least one arm and hand to steer and operate the control levers. Advantages of the scooter compared to the W/C are: narrower width, swivel seat, and a sportier look. Sliding transfers are possible if you request an armrest model that slips down even with the seat or swings out of the way. Though motorized scooters can be disassembled for transportation, and lifts have been designed to place the heavier parts in a car, you may still need some help getting the scooter in and out of the car. As with a motorized W/C, it is best to try the various scooters before purchasing one.

A W/C that cannot be operated independently is the Companion Chair. This chair is intended to be pushed by a companion and is a very narrow 20.5 inches (seat width is 17 inches), making it easy to maneuver in restaurants, theaters, and other crowded areas that may have narrow passageways. When the footplates are removed, the chair folds to a compact 27 by 23¾ by 8 inches. The arms are fixed, so standing is required when getting in and out of the chair.

Testing by the physical therapist or the occupational therapist and the prescription of a physiatrist will help ensure that you get the W/C and accessories matched to your needs.

WHEN DOORWAYS AND STEPS ARE A PROBLEM

Replacing door hinges with offset hinges will increase the opening 1.5 to 2 inches because the door will swing completely out of the opening. Door saddles (a raised strip of wood or marble where the floors of two rooms or a hallway and a room meet) should be removed and the space between the two floors made level if door saddles interfere with mobility.

A few steps can be ramped if there is room. For every inch in step height, the ramp should be 10 to 12 inches long for a person in a wheelchair to be able to push up the ramp. A platform (5 foot width, 3 foot length is recommended) at the top of the ramp will enable a person in a wheelchair to unlock and open a door. Mechanical devices, such as porch lifts, lower a wheelchair on a platform from the porch to street level; in the house, stair lifts carry a seated person up and down a straight or curved flight of stairs. These are expensive, and whenever possible a single-level dwelling should be sought.

CAR HAND CONTROLS

Car hand controls have given many people the freedom to drive wherever they wish, despite weakness in their legs. If you have good vision and hand function, hand controls can be installed in cars with automatic transmissions. This enables you to operate the brake and gas pedal safely through mechanical attachments. The installation does not interfere with foot operation so the car can still be driven by other family members.

GRAB BARS

If you have difficulty walking, you may want or need the additional security of grab bars attached to the wall or a lifeguard rail attached to the tub. Grab bars are tubular stainless steel sections mounted into wall support studs. Some are vinyl-covered for better grip and less heat absorption.

Grab bars can be mounted in any configuration: horizontal, vertical, diagonal, L-shaped, etc. A space the width of a clenched fist should exist between the grab bar and the wall to permit quick release and regrasp of the bar. If you are installing the bars yourself, follow the manufacturer's directions exactly; otherwise have them installed professionally. *Never, never* use towel racks, soap dishes, door knobs, etc. for support in the bathroom. These fixtures were not designed to support your body weight. Install a grab bar.

A lifeguard rail is also tubular stainless steel but in the configuration of an inverted U that can be securely attached by suction cups to the tub itself to provide a sure handhold.

A secure mat or nonslip treads are a must in the bathtub.

BATHING

A tub bench or shower chair used in conjunction with grab bars or a lifeguard rail may be helpful if stepping over the tub rim is no problem, but getting to the bottom of the tub and up again is difficult. The tub bench or shower chair permits bathing, more often showering, while seated. *Test the water temperature* to avoid burns; an inexpensive thermometer may be taped to the inside of a tub, and thermometers or thermostats which attach to the shower head are available. The water temperature should not exceed 100°F.

A transfer tub bench, with back support, is the safest solution when you cannot safely step over the tub rim (usually about 17 inches high). The simplest model transfer tub bench is a solid platform that extends across the tub, secured by two height-adjustable legs with attached suction cups inside the tub and two legs outside the tub. A grab bar along the wall may be desirable to assist sitting stability or standing.

Shower doors do not permit enough room for the transfer tub bench and transferring. Shower doors must be replaced by a shower curtain. Transferring to the bench involves a sliding transfer from a W/C, then lifting the legs over the tub rim; or if walking aids are used, it involves sitting on the bench and then lifting the legs over the rim. An occupational therapist, physical therapist, or other rehabilitation specialist should work with you until you feel secure doing the transfer. (If you use a W/C, the seat should be the same height as the transfer tub bench. If the bench is higher, it may be necessary to place a board under the W/C cushion or to add another cushion when making this transfer. Check with your therapist.)

Your feet should reach the bottom of the tub when seated on the transfer tub bench, which may not be the case if you have an old-style footed or raised tub, or if you are very short. A smaller bench or block of wood (sanded and sealed with polyurethane to prevent splinters) with attached suction cups may be placed in the tub to rest your feet on.

A more elaborate model, the padded transfer tub bench, is constructed of padded slats, to ensure water drainage into the tub; it also has a high back with one attached armrest (available on either the right or left side). An attached smaller bench extends about 12 inches beyond the tub, making transfers easier.

The easiest way to bathe while seated on a transfer tub bench is with a flexible shower hose (often sold in department stores for shampooing hair). This handheld shower unit can be attached by a bracket anywhere on the bathroom wall within convenient reach. More elaborate models provide an on/off switch as part of the hand-held unit and an optional diverter valve that permits conventional use of the shower head or tub spout.

A much more expensive alternative to the transfer tub bench is the bath lift. Powered by water pressure, this bath seat rises above the tub rim, swivels for transfers, then lowers to the bottom of the tub. Again, a therapist should be consulted to evaluate if you can safely transfer to the bath lift and independently manage the con-trolling levers (unfortunately placed behind or beneath the seat).

If you cannot transfer to any type of tub bench, a patient lifter may be attached to the tub rim to lift you from a W/C into the tub. You may prefer that a hammock-style chair, designed for this pur-pose and secured with front leg suction cups, be placed in the tub for more comfortable positioning.

SHOWERING

A shower chair or a fold-down bath seat fastened to the wall and a diagonal or L-shaped grab bar for stability when sitting or standing provide safety if you use a walking aid or tire easily while standing in the shower. A largish shower stall (with shower curtain, not a door) will accomodate a transfer tub bench, which measures ap-proximately 26 by 18 inches, for W/C sliding transfers. If there is adequate space to approach the shower in a wheeled shower chair, it may be possible to ramp the shower entrance so that a shower or commode chair can be rolled in.

Bathing or showering may be made easier by a long-handled sponge (some even hold the soap) to wash hard-to reach places, a wash mitt (eliminates the need to hold a wash cloth), and an octopus suction holder (tiny suction cups on both sides of a flat rubber disc firmly hold soap, shampoo bottles, etc. to the tub rim or shower shelf).

TOILETTING

The conventional toilet seat is often too low (about 15 to 17 inches) but can be altered with a removable or quickly installed raised toilet seat (also available with a padded seat) to increase the height 4 to 7 inches. If more assistance is needed when lowering to or rising from the toilet seat, grab bars may be placed on the wall alongside the toilet, or an easily installed toilet frame may be used on one or both sides.

Although a raised toilet seat is the easiest and quickest way to increase the height of the toilet seat, the entire fixture may be raised on a platform, or a wall-hung toilet may be installed. A wall-hung toilet has the additional advantage that it does not take up floor space and permits a closer approach by a W/C.

An electronically powered bidet unit, attached to an existing toilet, provides an easy way to cleanse yourself after toiletting if hand coordination problems make using tissue difficult or if weakness limits arm motion.

USING THE BATHROOM SINK

An open area below the bathroom sink, high enough to clear your knees, will allow you to sit comfortably at the sink. *To prevent burns, the hot water pipe and drainage pipe must be insulated.* A single-lever faucet may be more difficult to control, if you have tremors, than a faucet operated by two paddle-shaped handles. An extra shelf below a high medicine cabinet will hold frequently used items within easy reach, and a mirror on a flexible or extension arm can be positioned anywhere you need it. If it is impossible or very uncomfortable to use the sink in a small bathroom, consider placing toiletry items and a small mirror near the kitchen sink, which may be more accessible.

SHAMPOOING

Shampooing is probably easiest when showering or bathing with a flexible shower hose. If your hair must be washed while you are confined to bed, an inflatable shampoo basin will support your head in sudsy water and allow rinse water to drain away through a tube to a bedside container.

SHAVING

An electric razor is safest for shaving if you have tremors. Some reduction of tremors may be achieved by stabilizing your head against a headrest, grasping with your free hand the wrist of the hand holding the razor while keeping your elbows close to your body. A lightweight 1- to 2-lb wrist weight on the hand holding the razor may give additional stability. A razor holder (a strap attaches the electric razor securely to the palm of the hand) will prevent the razor from accidentally slipping from your grip.

ORAL HYGIENE

A built-up handle toothbrush or electric toothbrush may be easier to handle than a conventional one. If tremors are a problem, try the stabilization techniques suggested above.

USING THE KITCHEN

The goal of a functional kitchen is to help you save time and energy while enjoying meal preparation. This can be achieved through the careful selection of appliances, their placement, and the use of "kitchen gadgets" and techniques. If you are lucky enough to have the opportunity to completely redesign your kitchen, a U-shaped or L-shaped kitchen with unbroken counter space is the easiest within which to work. The major appliances should be placed in the following order: refrigerator, sink, and stove/oven, with counter space between them. This enables you to take food from the refrigerator, wash or prepare it at the sink and counter space, then move it to the stove or oven for cooking or baking.

All food preparation can be done while seated (with some accommodations in your environment), which will greatly reduce fatigue. You may choose to use one or more strategically placed sturdy kitchen stools with a backrest and footrest, a chair on casters, or a wheelchair. When a wheelchair or standard-height chair is used, counter space is generally too high for comfortable work; an extra cushion may be all that is necessary to increase the height—but check with your doctor or therapist to make sure your stability in the wheelchair is not at risk with the additional height. The most often recommended counter space height is 30 to 32 inches (27 inches for mixing). Determine the most comfortable height for you by working at a few different heights. This can be tested in the training kitchen of a rehabilitation center. If lowering the counter space is not possible, consider a wheeled table, drop-leaf table, or fold-down table hinged to the wall where it could conveniently serve as a work surface. If you are seated at the work surface, you will need knee room underneath. Knee room can sometimes be created under a counter by removing cabinet doors.

Once you have found a comfortable work height, determine how far you can easily reach forward, upward, and downward. Within the span of this reach is where most commonly used cookware and foodstuffs should be stored.

Organize cooking utensils according to their usage and near where they will be used: salad preparation items together between the refrigerator and sink, mixing and baking items together near the oven, skillet near the stove, and teakettle near the sink if you fill it with water directly from the sink, or on the stove if you fill it with a hose extension from the sink. Duplication, where needed, of frequently used items (measuring spoons, small mixing bowl, knife) will prevent traversing the kitchen several times during food preparation. Items bought in bulk or large containers are easier to manage when they are transferred to smaller cannisters. Generally, lightweight cannisters are best if you have weakness; heavy cannisters are best if you have tremors.

Maximize Storage Space

When you have determined your comfortable reach when seated or standing, consider the following, which may be purchased or built inexpensively, to maximize the storage space available to you.

Counterspace: A pull-out platform at the back of the counter rolls appliances within easy reach. Vertical dividers (for cookie sheets, muffin tins, etc.) can be placed at the back of the counter.

Kitchen cabinets: A revolving shelf unit (turntable) puts more items within reach. An added shelf or pull-out basket beneath the upper cabinets utilizes this empty space. A false back wall (or very large, little-used items placed on the back of the shelf) will keep items from being pushed back into the cabinet, beyond reach. When lower cabinet doors are removed, open shelf space is created. Drawers and pull-out bins can be added. If the shelves are removed, sliding racks with hooks, from which to hang pots, can be installed.

Drawers: A too-deep drawer can be raised with a false bottom. Vertical dividers in a deep drawer help store baking pans, etc. without stacking. A shallow drawer with diagonal dividers (tilted about 30° away from you) will hold canned goods so the labels are easily read.

Wallspace: Extra shelves or a pegboard with hooks for utensils utilizes empty wall space.

Closets: Narrow shelves with a lip or guard on the back of the closet door will hold cleaning items or canned goods. (Stronger hinges may be needed.) When the closet is too small to enter or maneuver within, consider a set of shelves on a dolly which pulls completely out of the closet, bringing everything within reach. The shelves should have a restraining lip, or guard, so items do not slip off. A mechanical reacher for *lightweight* items (a pudding box, not a can of vegetables) can increase the storage space that is accessible.

No matter what the design of your kitchen, you will be using a sink and certain basic types of appliances: a refrigerator, stove, and oven.

Refrigerator

The refrigerator door should open so that it does not block counter space. This way food taken from the refrigerator can be placed directly on the counter. If the door blocks the counterspace, a wheeled cart is useful for holding the food and can be pushed to the work area where the food is prepared.

Refrigerator shelves can be arranged so that the heaviest food is stored at the height that is easiest for you to reach when transferring food to the counterspace, or level with a wheelchair lapboard or wheeled cart. A revolving (turntable) unit on one or more shelves brings more food within reach at the front of the shelf.

Adding shelves in the freezer will prevent stacking too many items, which then become difficult to see and to reach. If the freezer is too deep to reach items in the back, water-filled plastic bottles placed in the back of the freezer will freeze and reduce the energy required to maintain the freezer temperature, as well as prevent stored items from being pushed to the back of the freezer beyond reach. A self-defrosting unit will save you a great deal of effort.

If your refrigerator/freezer does not have an automatic ice cube maker, carrying a half-full ice cube tray to the freezer is easier, as is placing trays in the freezer and filling them with fresh water from a plastic squeeze bottle.

The Sink

A shallow sink with the drain at a rear corner (to give more knee room when seated) is the easiest at which to work. A rubber mat at the bottom reduces breakage. A too-deep sink can be raised by a wood slat platform built to fit your sink, or a commercially available houseware item may work in your sink.

To prevent burns while seated at the sink, the bottom of the sink, hot water pipes, and drain should be covered with insulation. (This is important especially if you have decreased sensation and might not be aware if your leg were resting against a very hot surface.)

A retractable spray hose is useful not only for rinsing dishes in the drying rack but for filling pans with water on the stove, or filling pans on the counter and sliding them to the stove. Faucet handles may need an extension for you to reach them easily, or you may be able to replace them with large paddle-shaped handles (easier to manage with tremors) or a one-lever handle (easier to manage with one hand if your hands are weak). Brushes that attach to the sink by suction cups remain steady while you scrub glasses or silverware against them with one hand.

Cooking and Baking

A conventional range/oven combination may require a person to work sideways if he or she is seated. The controls may not be easy to reach, and the broiler may be so low that it is dangerous to reach for food there. The range/oven combination is easier to work at if immediately to one side there is counter space to serve as a work area and lower cabinets which can be removed to provide knee room for the seated person. The oven shelves should be kept clean so they will slide part-way out when removing food from the oven; long barbecue tongs can be used to reach food in the broiler. Still, for many people the counter work space and burners are too high to work at comfortably, and the broiler will almost certainly be too low to reach for cleaning.

One alternative is to replace the conventional range/oven with a lower self-cleaning wall oven with side opening door, and to sink parallel burners into a lowered counter space. Burners should be in a row so it will not be necessary to reach over a hot front burner to use a rear burner. You may prefer a wall oven with a front opening door that can be used as a shelf when removing food.

Another (less expensive) alternative is to use smaller appliances, such as a self-cleaning toaster oven/broiler or microwave oven, and an immersible electric skillet. An advantage of the microwave oven is that dishes remain cool while the food is being heated. Most recipes can be prepared in these smaller appliances, and they may be much easier to use if you are preparing food for only one or two people. Other applicances that may be useful are a coffee maker, a hot-pot for boiling water, a slow cooker, a mixer, and a blender or food processor.

When choosing an appliance, make sure the controls are easy to reach and manipulate, and that you can disassemble and reassemble the various parts for cleaning. Some controls can be built up by attaching a larger knob or lever, making it easier to grasp. Difficult-to-read temperature settings can sometimes be marked over a larger area of the appliance with bright, heat-resistant paint. It is wisest to choose only those appliances you use regularly, so storage space is not taken up by little-used items, and meal clean-up does not involve washing every appliance in the kitchen.

The addition of several appliances to a kitchen may draw too much power from the available outlets. An electrician can determine if you need another electrical line to the kitchen and can install a heavy-duty outlet box with extra outlets and a circuit breaker for safety.

Safety Techniques

1. Wear long, heat-resistant oven mitts when removing food from the oven.

2. Never lift hot food or liquid across your body.

3. *To light a gas burner or oven:* Place a lighted wooden match near the gas outlet, then turn on the gas. Alternatively, use a flint lighter which creates a spark when the handles are squeezed together (look for this item at camping stores).

Cutting Food

1. A serrated knife is easier to control than one with a straight blade.

2. A rocker knife with a curved blade or one-handed food chopper is used with one hand.

3. Some food is easier to cut with kitchen shears than with a knife.

4. If you use an electric knife, choose a cordless model.

5. To peel vegetables use an (old-fashioned) vegetable peeler with two floating blades, rather than a knife.

Transferring Hot Liquids and Foods

1. Ladle rather than pour hot liquids from a pan.
2. A baster will remove a small amount of hot liquid.
3. To remove food (vegetables, pasta, etc.) from boiling water: Boil the food in a steamer or deep-fry basket, which can be lifted out of the pan.

Frying Food

1. Choose long utensils.
2. Use barbecue tongs to turn food.
3. Wear a flame- and heat-retardant barbecue (or high school chemistry) apron.

Stabilization Techniques and Devices

1. A damp cloth sponge prevents a bowl from slipping.
2. Double suction cup holders hold a bowl firmly.
3. A cutting board with two nails in the center holds food steady.
4. A pan stabilizer attaches to the range by suction cups and limits movement of the pan.
5. A mixing bowl holder holds the bowl for mixing then tilts for pouring.
6. Kitchen gadgets are available in housewares departments and from self-help catalogs. The list is endless; here are just a few many people have found helpful:
   a. Plastic grater that fits into its own bowl.
   b. Whisk and eggbeaters operated by a downward pushing motion.
   c. One-hand flour-sifter with squeeze handle.
   d. Pizza roller for small amounts of pastry dough.
   e. One-hand rolling pin.
   f. Pastry blender (easy to grasp and use with one hand).
   g. Zim jar opener.
   h. Giant pop bottle opener.

i. Self-wringing sponge mop. (If your are using it from a seated position, saw the handle off at a convenient length, about 30 inches or so.)

j. Long-handled dust pan.

k. Plastic washtub on casters.

7. Some aids that may prove helpful when eating are:

a. Built-up handles to make thin utensils easier to grasp (a foam hair curler placed over the utensil handle may work well).

b. A rocker knife for one-handed cutting.

c. A plastic tumbler with lid and hole for a straw, or a vac-u-flow cup with lid and built-in straw prevent liquids from spilling. (When drinking hot liquids, use a terry cloth coaster that fits around the bottom of the cup.)

d. Some people have found that 1- to 2-lb wrist weights help steady tremors when they are eating.

THE BEDROOM

A bedroom that is easy to move around in, where everything is comfortably placed, may require only a little rearranging and few modifications. To make transfers easier, the bed height can be lowered by shortening the legs of the bed frame, or raised by using leg extenders or wooden blocks (with at least a 3-foot deep cutout to securely hold the leg). A backrest or several pillows layered to support the shoulders and head and an over-bed table are useful if you spend much time in bed. (If you use a wheelchair, choose an over-bed table with a base that fits around a wheelchair.) An adjustable bed, manual or motorized, may be the best solution if you are most comfortable in bed. If it is difficult for you to change position in bed, a foam "egg crate" mattress placed directly under the sheet will reduce the pressure of the mattress against your body. If your skin is sensitive to pressure, or you have ever had a skin breakdown (pressure sore), your doctor will recommend one of the many other pressure-reducing/pressure-distributing mattresses.

A bedside table to hold water, a telephone, buzzer, or intercom, and other items, as well as a good light source, should be within convenient reach of the bed. "Goose neck" holders are available to hold a telephone receiver in one position, and large extensions to fit over both rotary and pushbutton phones make dialing easier. Telephone units with a memory eliminate dialing frequently used numbers. Simple adaptations can also be added to the lighting fixture if it is difficult to use: a knob or curtain ring at the end of a pull cord makes it easier to grasp, a large lamp switch extension lever fits over small lamp switches, and an extender brings too-high wall switches within reach. Recently on the market are remote control boxes that enable you to turn on/off a number of electrical devices (such as lights, television, and air conditioner). On/off control switches are also available on extension cords—just be sure the cord is well out of the way (perhaps taped to the baseboard) to prevent tripping over it or becoming entangled in it.

The most comfortable storage height, whether standing or seated, is between shoulder and knee height. If drawers at this height stick, try a silicone spray made to prevent sticking, or see if they can be refitted with glides. If the drawers are difficult to open because two handles are widely spaced, try pulling on a wide ribbon tied between the two handles, or replacing them with one large centered handle. A lowered closet rod will accommodate shirts, folded slacks, jackets, skirts, and dresses folded at the waist.

Some aids that may be helpful when dressing are:

1. Placing your foot on a stepstool when tying your shoes if it is difficult to reach your shoes on the floor.

2. Elastic shoe laces (your feet can slip into the shoe without retying each time) or Velcro closures which must be sewn on at a shoe repair shop.

3. A long-handled shoe horn.

4. A button aid that slips through the button hole, attaches around the button and pulls it through the hole, using only one hand.

5. A stocking aid that holds pantyhose or socks open, allowing you to slip your foot into the sock and pull the sock up.

6. Velcro to replace difficult-to-manage hooks and eyes, snaps, zippers, etc.

There are many other aids available to help in the performance of these and other functions. The need for them must be carefully worked out depending on how much reduction in functional ability has occurred, and if they can be used effectively. The cost/benefit ratio must be considered seriously so that the greatest benefit to function will be achieved at the lowest possible cost. In this respect, consultation with skillful occupational and physical therapists will guarantee that the most favorable ratio will be achieved. To extend one's range and therefore one's horizons, and to improve one's capacity to perform the activities of daily living are major contributions to the quality of living. For many, not much of the foregoing will be necessary, but for the few who need them, they will help liberate you from a constricted life style.

9

Nursing Care

Nancy J. Holland, Phyllis Wiesel-Levison, and
Margaret McDonnell

The vast majority of individuals with multiple sclerosis require hospitalization only infrequently. However, there are times when it is necessary to enlist the help of a nurse in the home. In these cases it is useful to understand the nurse's role and how he or she can be of the most assistance.

One of the nurse's most important functions is to interpret technical terms the MS person and family may hear discussed. Once understood, these medical words are less fearsome. The nurse can also explain the disease process and what to expect from it, as well as provide a better understanding about the various symptoms and what causes them, the tests the MS patient sometimes has to undergo, and finally the treatments prescribed.

Although the nurse has the potential of providing these services, much of the delivery depends on the inquisitiveness of the patient and his or her family. It is best for the individual and family to approach the problem as a modern consumer would who is buying an appliance or a new car—they are, after all, consumers of health care and should adopt a direct and questioning attitude. When the patient has adopted this attitude, he or she has assumed some control over the situation, which in itself can create a more optimistic atmosphere.

PHILOSOPHY OF HEALTH CARE

The philosophy of modern "health care" views health as the optimal level of function and well-being within the possible limitations imposed by a physical or emotional impairment. From this viewpoint, a person with congenital deafness can be healthy, as can a person with MS. For the individual with MS, an important component of health is the absence of disease activity, that is, a remission (disappearance) of symptoms or a stabilization of the situation, where there is no further progression of symptoms. However, even when this is not the current situation, health as the highest possible level of well-being is still a goal.

A team approach to the individual in need of medical help fosters comprehensive care and a holistic view of the patient. This means that he or she is viewed as a unique individual who functions in a particular way within his family and the community. This approach can be difficult to maintain given the scope of services which may be required, the number of health care providers involved, and the fact that geographically scattered agencies are called on to address assorted needs. The nurse often assumes the role of coordinator of these services.

GOOD HEALTH IS POSSIBLE

Implicit in the concept of health is the idea of freedom from illness, which for the MS person means good general health as well as an absence of disease-related complications.

Nutrition

Maintaining good health starts with good and proper nutrition. There are various aspects of nutrition that are important. It is essential to keep body weight stable. This is a very practical consideration. The MS individual may find it difficult to walk—and with excess weight it becomes even harder. Transferring from a wheelchair to the toilet or a car becomes a major feat for the obese person. Conversely, the very thin, wheelchair-bound person who has insufficient "padding" to protect against pressure and potential skin breakdown (bed sores, pressure sores) needs to increase caloric intake. Hence keeping the body at a reasonable weight is simply a matter of practicality.

The patient with inadequate nutrition may be less resistant to infection, and so a diet of nutritious foods is advised to attain the desired body weight.

Constipation may be a problem that is caused by inadequate fluid intake. In these cases increased bulk and more fluids should be added to the diet. Bran cereals are helpful, as are fresh and cooked fruits and vegetables, whole-grain bread, and prune juice.

Urinary tract infections are sometimes a problem for MS patients. Here certain dietary measures can be taken to increase the urinary acidity, which reduces this risk. Cranberry and prune juices promote an acidic urine and are therefore helpful in preventing urinary tract infections. Orange, grapefruit, and tomato juice have components in them that cause the urine to become just the opposite, alkaline, and so should be taken in limited amounts.

As in the general population, some individuals with MS may have other health problems such as diabetes or high blood pressure (hypertension). While diet is of major importance in controlling diabetes, the physician can recommend a dietary program which includes MS-related needs. Hypertension usually requires salt restriction. When diuretics (drugs to remove excess fluid from the body) are also needed, measures used to manage MS urinary problems might be readjusted in the MS patient. The doctor will probably redesign the drug-taking schedule. The nurse can assist with determining the necessary dietary changes, and help the MS person and family with meal planning which follows the individually prescribed diet.

Rest and Exercise

Good health requires an adequate balance between rest and physical activity. The proper balance varies for each individual, one having a need for more rest or sleep than another. The MS person must take care to maintain this delicate balance, since he or she may become easily fatigued. In addition, intolerance of heat and humidity may be a problem. It is believed that greater energy is required to transmit signals in the nervous system past the damaged myelin (the fatty material around the nerve that is damaged or destroyed in MS) than is needed when the nervous system is intact.

If this is true, then minimal physical activity may result in a disproportionate energy drain or sense of fatigue. Furthermore, anything which raises the body temperature may heighten this energy loss and/or accentuate any MS symptoms the person is experiencing.

When the MS person is easily fatigued or finds heat-sensitivity a problem, exercise (as range of motion exercises) must be carefully planned so as not to use up all the individual's energy, leaving little or none for other activities necessary to daily living such as work and socialization.

The visiting nurse or public health nurse agencies can often refer a physical therapist to plan a home program of exercise aimed at maintaining muscle strength and joint mobility while conserving energy for activities of daily living. The most highly recommended exercise is swimming because body temperature is not elevated and buoyancy in the water permits greater movement. Exercise may be done in an air-conditioned room which controls heat and humidity, so the body does not become overheated.

Rest periods to maximize energy during the day need to be carefully planned. MS individuals often have a high energy level during the morning but experience increasing fatigue in the afternoon hours. Recognizing this, a daily schedule can be planned with the more tiring or demanding activities scheduled for the morning hours. For example, the housewife may choose to shop early in the day when stores are less crowded and her energy level is higher. Light household chores and dinner preparation can then be done at a more leisurely pace in the afternoon, with a brief rest period or nap if needed. When low energy or a pattern of easy exhaustion is encountered, alternating activity with rest periods will usually improve overall function.

Nonexercise-related Body Temperature Elevation

Any individual's body temperature may increase when struck by "flu", a sore throat, or other infection. The increase may be very slight, but the person with MS may find that weakness worsens to the extent that a person who is normally ambulatory may not be able to walk. Fortunately, this worsening of symptoms is usually temporary, as it is after excessive exercise.

Corrective measures for this weakening effect are aimed at identifying and eliminating the cause of the fever when possible, as with a urinary tract or other infection, and at reducing the body temperature to normal. The doctor or nurse should always be called when this occurs. The temperature may be reduced by taking aspirin or Tylenol every 4 hours along with drinking cool fluids. The patient's temperature should be checked every 4 to 6 hours to make sure it is being lowered—that the treatment is working.

If the infection is severe (for instance if there is a possible severe urinary tract infection, pneumonia, or an infected pressure sore, or if the person is already very ill), the doctor may recommend hospitalization.

Hot baths or showers, steam from a hot stove or iron, or prolonged exposure to the sun may also temporarily elevate the body temperature. The first effect from this elevated body temperature may show up as slight blurring of the vision or a general feeling of weakness.

When a person with MS realizes that he or she is subject to heat intolerance (from any source), exposure to any situation in which the body becomes overheated should be avoided.

SYMPTOMS DIRECTLY RELATED TO MS

The person with MS can, at any given time, experience symptoms of the disease. Because this is so, it is well to recognize the symptoms and to know how to alleviate them.

A symptom is a perceptible change in the body or its functions which indicates disease. Symptoms of MS vary in severity, duration, and their effect on the individual's daily function. Their significance in terms of the course of the disease and in terms of the individual's response to therapy also is quite different from one patient to another. Given the diversity of potential symptoms, the person with MS may find it difficult to sort out which symptoms are MS related and which are not. In this situation the nurse or physician should be contacted to help resolve the question and to prescribe treatment since symptomatic treatment may be available. Moreover, such a change may signify a point at which more aggressive therapy should be considered.

Sensory symptoms—numbness, tingling, a sense of constriction as if a tight band had been applied, and vague, peculiar skin sensations—tend to be temporary. They may "come and go" for a number of months. Some sensory disturbances are more troubling, however, such as burning or pain along the course of a nerve. These are also temporary and may be controlled by medication such as carbamazepine (Tegretol) or phenytoin sodium (Dilantin). Although sensory symptoms cause discomfort, they are considered benign in that they do not affect the overall prognosis of MS.

Visual symptoms—blurring, double vision, pain in the eye, or "blind spots"—also tend to be temporary and do not signify a serious course of MS. These symptoms may be alleviated more rapidly if steroids are administered, and so a short course of oral prednisone is sometimes prescribed by the physician.

Motor symptoms are those which interfere with movement. In the MS patient these are seen most frequently as leg weakness. Coordination problems include imbalance while walking, involuntary hand movements, and jumping of the eyes. Although motor and coordination symptoms are often resistant to treatment, some therapies are available. These are described in Chapter 7.

Symptoms caused by bladder or bowel dysfunction must be reported to the doctor, who can prescribe various measures to relieve them. These therapy forms are discussed in Chapter 10. A small percentage of patients with advanced MS have more serious symptoms which are discussed later in this chapter.

When concern about a symptom is present, the MS person or family should contact the nurse, who can then help determine the proper course of action to pursue. This may be a visit to the doctor or local emergency room, or simply reassurance that no action is needed. Again, the nurse's role is to provide information needed for better understanding of the disease and its manifestations so all concerned can better follow the most beneficial course of action.

SKIN PROTECTION

A person's skin condition rarely is a topic for conversation. For the MS person, however, it is of prime importance to understand how the skin acts as a protective agent, how to recognize and prevent potential problems, and the relevance of good hygiene and a well-balanced diet.

Skin constitutes the outer covering of the entire body. There are several layers of this covering which protect body tissues from outside harm. Any break in the skin through which bacteria may enter is a potential source of infection. Such breaks may be caused by irritation or by rubbing a particular area for prolonged periods. In addition, direct contact with moisture, as may occur with urinary leakage, may also precipitate skin breakdown. However, the major threat for susceptible MS patients is skin breakdown due to pressure.

People with MS who have sensory deficits are candidates for skin breakdown, since danger signals indicating too much pressure exists are not felt (or only slightly so). Pressure on a particular body area for any length of time, without the person moving or changing position to reduce the pressure, decreases the blood flow to that spot. This reduces the oxygen and nutrients necessary for tissue health. If an area lacks these components for a long period of time, the tissue may die *(necrosis)*. This process may begin after only an hour of continuous pressure and is much more difficult to reverse than to prevent.

The result of such reduced circulation is a pressure sore (also known as a bedsore or a decubitus ulcer). It usually occurs over bony prominences (sacrum, ankles, elbows) and other pressure points (heels). The earliest sign of this sore is a reddened area that progresses to a superficial skin blister which subsequently opens. Alternatively, the sore may start as a blackened, soft area under the skin. Fluid may ooze from the sore, and the affected area may increase in width and depth. Once the problem is recognized, treatment should be initiated. Specific treatment is discussed later in this section.

Pressure sores may also be caused by a device such as a leg or hand brace that is improperly fitted or poorly padded. They can appear on the person confined to a wheelchair or one who is sitting all day in an office. It is extremely important to keep in mind that when there is a decrease in sensation one will not feel the damaging pressure, and so the sore will be discovered only after harmful effects have occurred. The key to good skin care is thus awareness and prevention.

If the wheelchair-bound person is able to stand, he should do so every hour for about 1 to 3 minutes. An excellent way to relieve pressure on the sacrum and tuberosities (buttocks) is to lock the wheelchair, hold onto its sides or to a table in front of the wheelchair, and then stand. The person unable to stand may lock the chair and do pushups by grasping the arms of the chair. Both of these exercises relieve pressure on the buttocks and sacrum and allows improved blood flow to that area. A good seat cushion is an essential preventative item for the wheelchair-bound person.

Swelling and/or discoloration of the ankles and feet usually indicates poor circulation in the lower extremities. Blood flow from the feet and legs is normally aided by pumping action of the calf muscles, and so decreased activity of the leg muscles results in an accumulation of fluid. This may predispose to skin breakdown. For this reason the wheelchair-bound person should occasionally elevate his or her legs on the wheelchair foot rests or place them on a chair or sofa to reduce swelling. Actively or passively moving the legs will also help circulation, as will "kicking" or having the legs raised and lowered by another person. Support stockings may also be helpful.

Severely disabled people with MS may easily develop pressure sores. In order to avoid this, the bed-ridden MS person should do additional exercises. One such exercise may be done as follows:

Turn from side to side or onto the abdomen every 2 hours, even during the night. The MS person may be able to turn independently; alternatively, he may help the caretaker turn him by grasping the side rails and pulling himself over, or by using an overhead trapeze (attached to the bed). Pillows should be positioned in strategic places

(a) for comfort, (b) to prevent any unintentional change in position, and (c) to avoid pressure over a bony prominence. When lying on the side, one pillow is placed between the lower legs to separate the knees and ankles, and one behind the back to provide support. After turning, it is wise to massage the area that had been laid on with a skin lotion or cream to help restore circulation. Creased sheets should also be smoothed at this time.

An air or water mattress and sheepskin heel and elbow protectors are also useful measures for preventing pressure sores. In addition, a daily bath (in bed or tub) is needed, as is good care of the nails. These should be cut to prevent the patient from scratching, which might result in a subsequent break in the skin. It is also extremely important to ensure adequate nutrition so as to keep the body tissues healthy and less prone to breakdown.

Prevention of skin breakdown is an important goal because the consequences of pressure sores are significant. When a sore occurs:

1. Long periods of immobility are required to promote healing, as the absence of any pressure and exposure to the air are needed for healing.

2. Tissue damage can extend to underlying skeletal structures, resulting in bone infection (osteomyelitis) which tends to be chronic and poorly controlled.

3. Extensive muscle/skin grafting may be needed because of the generally poor blood circulation to areas of potential skin breakdown. (Poor circulation interferes with the healing process.)

4. Infection rapidly develops after skin breakdown and damage to the tissues underneath. This may proceed to "blood poisioning" (septicemia) and may be life-threatening.

Treatment of Pressure Sores

At the first sign that a pressure sore is forming, measures should be initiated to prevent worsening. If any area on the body is excessively red, massage it with a skin lotion and change the individual's position. If there is a small break in the skin, it should be treated immediately. The area must be kept clean, dry, and without pressure. The first step is to cleanse the affected skin with povidone iodine (Betadine) solution, a brown antiseptic which may stain linens but is readily removed from the skin with soap and water. Betadine is applied by saturating a gauze pad with the solution and then dabbing the area of skin breakdown. This will cleanse the area, deter infection, and help dry the sore. It is not necessary to place a bandage or gauze pad on the spot unless the person will be sitting on the sore for any length of time or it is in an area where there may be contact with feces. A blow-type hair dryer may be used to dry the sore, in conjunction with the Betadine; if the dryer is used, blow warm (not hot) air on the sore at a distance of approximately 10 inches. A topical powder, Thymol Iodide, may be lightly dusted over the site to further dry the sore and avoid infection. Vaseline or other lubricating creams should be avoided at this time, although these may be helpful if the skin has not yet broken.

The nurse should be notified when any skin breakdown is observed. She or he will evaluate the area and advise the patient or caretaker about the appropriate treatment. In some situations a small piece of gauze may be needed to keep the skin separated, preventing the area from closing on the surface until the underlying tissues have healed. If dead (necrotic) tissue is present, it may need to be gradually cleared away by applying a special enzyme ointment. In some cases the sore seems to be superficial even though the actual damage has progressed to some depth or infection has already started. The nurse may advise immediate examination by a physician, and in any event will inform him or her about the status of the pressure sore. The nurse should then continue to monitor the condition of the pressure sore until healing has taken place and will help to obtain whatever supplies are needed for care.

In all cases, pressure must be kept off the affected area. Exposure to the air is also advised as much as possible. When the sore is located on or near the buttocks, the person will be required to remain in bed and off the sore for long periods each day. This may be distressing to the individual who is normally active, but it is essential if more serious, even life-threatening injury is to be avoided.

If the decubitus continues to worsen (becomes wider, deeper, changes color to black, or drains blood, clear fluid, or pus), more aggressive treatment may be required that calls for hospitalization. During this time, the wound may be cleansed in a whirlpool-type bath (Hubbard tank) in which most of the body is immersed. This also helps to improve circulation to the impaired tissues. If the person cannot control urinary flow, a Foley catheter may be inserted to keep the wound dry and promote healing. If the sore has become infected, antibiotics are likely to be administered to prevent a more serious infection from developing.

This is often sufficient treatment to help heal the wound. While in the hospital the MS person may be placed on a special bed, such as a circoelectric bed, an Egerton net bed, a sand bed, or a water bed or mattress. All of these are designed to reduce the pressure on the sore and promote healing.

A pressure sore rarely requires surgery to close it, but if all else fails this may be recommended. Dead tissue may need to be removed before healing can take place. Circulation is poor in areas where pressure sores usually form, and so it may be necessary to have a skin or muscle graft from an area that has a good blood supply. The area where skin has been removed generally heals without any further difficulty, as does the grafted area.

PASSIVE EXERCISE

Some individuals with MS cannot move one or more of their arms or legs because of weakness, incoordination, or spasticity (muscle stiffness or tightness). When this situation exists, the limb(s) must be passively exercised, either by the MS person or someone else, in order to maintain full movement of that joint (elbow, wrist, knee, ankle). The arm or leg is moved through all the positions that would be possible with a normal limb. All joints need to be moved. In the case of an affected arm, the shoulder, elbow, wrist, and fingers should be manipulated; for the leg it is the hip, knee, ankle, and toes. These exercises, called passive range of motion (PROM), should be done at least twice a day. Bathing and dressing are convenient times for this.

The purpose of the PROM exercises is to maintain full joint mobility, thereby avoiding painful and potentially dangerous contractures. A contracture is a "frozen joint" in which permanent changes in the joint prohibit return of movement. If contracture occurs, surgical correction is needed for mobility to be restored. The contracture interferes with activities of daily living, such as dressing. For example, it is difficult to put on a shirt or jacket if no movement in the shoulder is possible. When the MS person tries to move the frozen joint, he experiences severe pain. Furthermore, contracture means that skin surfaces are continuously in contact, which causes irritation, often resulting in skin breakdown with ulceration. Hygiene is also impaired by the joint immobility.

When spasticity contributes to limitation of movement, the extremity should be gently stretched. Most often the patient holds the leg or arm in a bent (flexed) position. It then needs to be slowly straightened (extended) in order to mobilize the joint.

It is important to keep the body and extremities moving so the circulation is maintained, as well as to prevent contractures and pressure sores. Turning from side to side and sitting up in a chair helps circulate the blood (oxygen and essential nutrients) throughout the body. This also avoids fluid collection in the lungs and so minimizes the possibility of lung congestion which may lead to pneumonia. Body movement also reduces the rate at which calcium is lost from the bones, thereby helping to decrease the incidence of stone formation in the urinary system.

It has thus become apparent that the benefits of getting the usually bedridden person into a chair are numerous. In addition to the advantages already discussed, the change of position increases comfort, facilitates eating and drinking, and increases the self-esteem of the person. To be able to sit up and be a part of family activities is a wonderful feeling and reduces the sense of isolation.

If needed, the very disabled person can be gotten out of bed by the use of a Hoyer lift or Trans-Aid. Both of these are hydraulic devices operated with very little effort on the part of the caretaker. Tub bathing may be accomplished at this time, as the use of the hydraulic lift makes the task easier. Bathing is very refreshing for the patient and maintains good body hygiene. Change of bedding and sheets are also done with greater ease while the person is out of bed. Wet or even creased sheets cause discomfort and may result in skin breakdown.

The various kinds of passive exercise which may be needed, depending on the MS patient's particular situation, are all useful in promoting comfort and mobility as well as preventing illness due to complications. The nurse can advise the patient and/or caretaker in the home when the need for some form of passive exercise has been identified.

Correction of Contractures

When joint mobility has become limited, it is necessary to identify if a contracture or merely a stiff joint is present.

A physician who specializes in rehabilitation (physiatrist) may make this determination by physical examination. In some cases the patient may require examination while under general anesthesia (in the hospital) so that an accurate diagnosis can be made.

If a contracture is present, surgical correction is necessary. When joint stiffness results from severely spastic muscles, a nerve block (injection of phenol into the nerve) may be necessary to relax the muscles and permit return of joint mobility. Whichever joint condition is present, a course of physical therapy is needed after the corrective measures in order to maximize restored joint mobility.

SAFETY MEASURES

One must be safe in his own environment in order to prevent unforeseen complications that may result from accidents or injuries. For the person with decreased sensation, special care is in order. For instance, the temperature of bath water must be checked with a thermometer or by the unaffected arm or leg. Otherwise scalding and serious burns may result because of the affected individual's diminished perception of extreme heat or cold.

Caution is also needed in the kitchen or when smoking cigarettes. Padded potholder mitts should be used for removing pots from the stove and baking dishes from the oven. Hot water bottles and heating pads should be avoided unless their use is directly supervised by an unimpaired individual.

Decreased sensory perception can also result in frostbite during cold weather or when storing food in a freezer. Warm clothing, including gloves should be worn during frigid weather, and oven mitts should be used when handling frozen food for any length of time.

Shoes need to be properly fitted as blisters can quickly develop without notice when sensation in the feet is impaired.

Accidental falls in the home are another potential danger. Throw rugs should be removed and grab bars installed where needed, as in the bathroom. The MS person should use some mobility aid—whether it is a cane, crutch, walker, or wheelchair—when appropriate. Three or more falls within a month suggest that the proper device is not being used or that the person needs additional training with the particular device.

These and other safety measures can be discussed with the nurse. When a particular problem area is identified, the nurse may refer an occupational or physical therapist for more extensive evaluation and recommendations. More detailed information on safety measures in the home is provided in Chapter 8.

The patient with urinary problems may have another source of potential injury—the catheter that stays inside the bladder (Foley catheter). This catheter is inserted through the urinary opening and is held in place by a small balloon inflated within the bladder. A sudden tug on the catheter may forcibly withdraw it from the bladder, causing internal injury as the inflated balloon exits from the body. This can be avoided by taping the catheter to the upper thigh of the female patient or to lower abdomen of the male patient using hypoallergenic tape.

MANAGING RENAL IMPAIRMENT

In rare instances, MS bladder dysfunction (neurogenic bladder) becomes a serious health problem. This happens when the kidney is damaged, and it is clearly a complication, rather than part of MS, as MS does not involve the kidneys directly. Urinary drainage from the kidney may need to be surgically diverted by means of a nephrostomy (Chapter 10). Urine then exits through an opening in the abdomen, bypassing the remainder of the urinary tract. When a kidney has been irreversibly damaged by prolonged "back-up" (reflux) of urine from the bladder or by repeated kidney infections (pyelonephritis), the kidney may need to be removed (nephrectomy). Following these surgical procedures (Chapter 10), meticulous care and monitoring of fluid balance is indicated because it is likely that the remaining kidney has also sustained some damage. The nurse can be called on to assist the patient and family in carrying out the individualized medical plan so that optimal function and comfort can be maintained.

DEALING WITH SWALLOWING DIFFICULTY

Impaired swallowing is a direct result of advanced MS and is not treatable by any currently known medical therapy. Mild dysfunction may be dealt with by dietary modifications aimed at maintaining adequate nutrition and preventing aspiration pneumonia. This complication occurs when food or fluid goes into the lungs rather than the stomach.

Fluids are frequently difficult to swallow, and so thicker forms such as milkshakes, jello, or sherbet may be eaten instead. Food which crumbles (toast, cake, potato chips) should be avoided. Small frequent meals are generally better tolerated than large meals, and soft food is more easily swallowed than solid food, which requires extensive chewing.

When swallowing is impaired to the extent that it is no longer safe to take food by mouth, a surgical procedure will be needed to create an alternate route for food and fluid intake. The two most common procedures are gastrostomy and esophagostomy.

With a gastrostomy, an opening is created in the stomach which is accessible through a tube in the abdomen. The tube is then changed by the nurse or physician every 4 tod 6 months. A gauze pad is cut from one edge to its center, placed around the gastrostomy tube, and held there by hypoallergenic tape. In some cases special skin care is needed, as when gastric juices irritate the skin or scar tissue develops. This should be discussed with the nurse.

An esophagostomy consists of an opening being made in the esophagus (the passageway which connects the mouth to the stomach) with access through an opening in the neck. Unlike the gastrostomy, no tube is left in place and skin problems are minimal because of the distance from the irritating gastric juices. Blenderized food and fluids are easily "fed" through either the gastrostomy or esophagostomy. Furthermore, the route for normal swallowing remains intact so that small amounts of desired foods may be taken by mouth to provide pleasure through the sense of taste.

OTHER COMPLICATIONS

Other complications may occur, such as pneumonia, but treatment is standard and not specific for MS. Individuals with advanced MS will require care in many or all activities of daily living. These measures are dealt with earlier in this and other chapters.

REHABILITATION

Rehabilitation is defined in *Stedman's Medical Dictionary* as "restoration, following disease, illness, or injury, of ability to function in a normal or near normal manner." In a broader view, rehabilitation includes all efforts to achieve optimal function in activities of daily living, within given limitations of the disease or disability. Many health professionals are involved in rehabilitation, notably physical and occupational therapists, rehabilitation counselors, nurses, social workers, and physicians who specialize in this field (physiatrists). All of these people are concerned with improving the patient's level of function and developing adaptive strategies to maximize the potential of each individual. The development of adaptive strategies is a helpful concept, as rehabilitation is a carefully formulated and continuously revised plan of action. For the person with MS this ongoing readjustment of goals and activities is essential, although very difficult. What is possible and desirable? This is the major question that must be answered before any rehabilitation effort is undertaken.

OVERCOMING FATIGUE

Determining the most suitable balance of rest and activity/exercise is the initial challenge in reducing easy fatigue as a disability. Other measures can also be advantageous, particularly those which reduce the amount of energy expended in mobility (getting from one place to another).

Most people with MS are ambulatory; some need no help whatsoever, whereas others require assistance. Assistive devices or techniques vary from holding onto walls (wall-walking) or onto another person for support to using a cane, crutches, or walker for stability. It is often a slow and painful process to accept an assistive device, as it is first necessary to acknowledge the loss of function. The goal is to view the mobility aid as an asset which expands the scope of possible activities and promotes safety from potentially serious falls, rather than as a symbol of disease progression. It is important to recognize that a sense of loss and sadness is bound to accompany increased difficulty in walking, while at the same time being able to accept the value of adopting whatever mobility aid is indicated.

For the struggling ambulatory person, a motorized chair such as a Scooter or Amigo is recommended. These vehicles are smaller than wheelchairs, easily maneuvered, and battery-operated. They resemble golf carts, and the components are easily taken apart so they can be transported in the trunk of a car. Sometimes it takes such strenuous efforts just to reach one's destination that the MS person has no energy left for what he set out to do. This struggle can be overcome with these motorized aids, which leave the person with enough energy to accomplish other tasks.

SUMMARY

For the person with MS, sickness—or deviation from general good health—occurs when disease-related complications have developed or when the MS progresses to an advanced, severely debilitating state. As with the focus on the prevention of illness, nursing care falls within the primary objective of health promotion. The treatment of complications is aimed at restoring the person with MS to his or her condition of health prior to the particular difficulty. When MS has progressed to an advanced state, the general goal remains the promotion of health to the optimal level possible within the disease limitations. This concept may be disconcerting for those who have trouble thinking of MS and health together. However, this orientation strives for a positive approach regarding what can be done, rather than a negative or hopeless outlook toward the person with MS who is sick because of primary or secondary effects of the disease.

Nursing care is administered not only by the professional nurse but by family members and other caretakers who strive to meet the physical and emotional needs of the person with MS. Although serious problems may be encountered, successful management of MS-related problems can be achieved by the cooperation of the patient, the family, and the individual providing nursing care services.

10

Bladder and Bowel Management

Nancy J. Holland and Arthur S. Abramson

Urinary symptoms are common in multiple sclerosis (MS), with as many as 80% of individuals affected at some time during the course of the disease. Bowel problems, especially constipation, also occur frequently. Symptoms in both of these areas are distressing and may interfere with personal, social, and vocational activities. Symptoms of bladder and bowel disorders, their meaning, and their treatment are discussed in this chapter. Understanding normal function, being able to relate symptoms to the actual physical impairment, and being aware of what can be expected from various treatments will help you identify problems and indications for seeking professional help. It will also help you to participate in your own bladder and bowel management.

DISORDERS OF URINARY FUNCTION

The individual with MS has a good chance of achieving average life expectancy if complications are avoided or minimized. Recurrent urinary tract infection, with its potential for kidney damage, is a major complication and presents an impediment to good health and longevity. The need to urinate frequently and suddenly without warning, and the loss of urinary control, inhibit socialization, interfere with job performance, and cause embarrassment in intimate circumstances (such as sexual activity). Feelings of self-esteem and enthusiasm to pursue rewarding experiences may be greatly diminished.

The hopeful aspect for persons with urinary disorders is that serious complications can be prevented and distressing symptoms relieved. However, some individuals become accustomed to these disorders and so they need to be reminded that dysfunction exists and be reassured that improvement is possible. Some ways that symptoms are rationalized are: "I wet myself because: (a) the front door key stuck; (b) we had to stop for a red light; (c) I had coffee that morning; (d) my kids tie up the bathroom." These excuses might be a reasonable way of dealing with an irreversible problem— but fortunately, bladder symptoms can be relieved. Acknowledgment that a problem exists is the first step and should be considered by anyone with a diagnosis of MS.

NORMAL BLADDER FUNCTION

A person with normal bladder function passes urine only four to six times within a 24-hour period. He can postpone urination until it is convenient, allowing him to sleep uninterruptedly; this ability also avoids "accidental urination."

The urinary bladder stores urine which is continuously produced by the kidneys and carried to the bladder through two small tubes called ureters (Fig. 1). When about 200 milliliters (ml), which is slightly less than a cup, has accumulated, the individual usually becomes aware of urine in the bladder. Contractions of the bladder, signaling a desire to urinate, are inhibited by the nervous system until 300 to 500 ml (roughly 1 to 2 cups) have collected. At this point, urination (also called voiding) is voluntarily initiated. For voiding to occur, the bladder contracts to expel urine through a thin tube called the urethra. At the same time, a valve-like muscle (the *sphincter*) in the urethra relaxes so the urine can easily pass. Thus when an adequate amount of urine is present, the bladder contracts, expelling all of the urine, and the sphincter relaxes, allowing the urine to flow out of the body. This all occurs automatically; but as bladder fullness can be sensed by the individual, emptying can be postponed by voluntarily contracting the sphincter until a more convenient time for voiding.

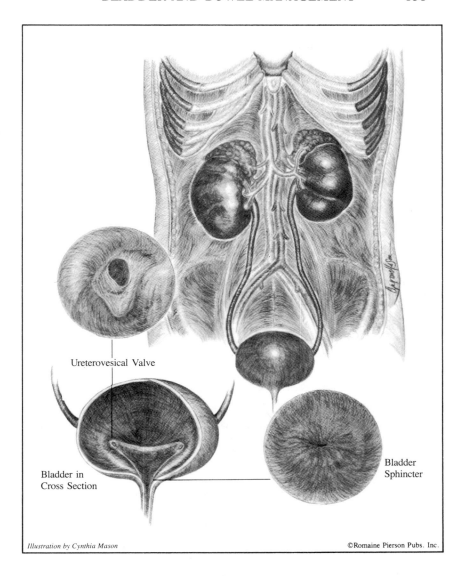

Ureterovesical Valve

Bladder in
Cross Section

Bladder
Sphincter

Illustration by Cynthia Mason   ©Romaine Pierson Pubs. Inc.

FIG. 1. Bladder anatomy.

PROBLEMS IN URINARY FUNCTION

Bladder dysfunction in MS is associated with spinal cord disease and is referred to as *neurogenic bladder*. It may produce the following symptoms:

Urgency. Once the desire to void is experienced, urination cannot be postponed until convenient. A toilet must always be in close proximity.

Frequency. The person must void more frequently than every 2 to 3 hours.

Hesitancy. Once at the toilet, the individual sometimes has difficulty initiating the flow of urine. This may occur despite the sense of "urgency."

Incontinence or enuresis. Passage of urine occurs before the toilet is reached (accidents). Loss of urinary control during sleep is called nocturnal enuresis.

Nocturia. The person is awakened by a need to urinate. This may occur one to five times a night.

Urinary tract infections or cystitis. Anyone may develop a urinary tract infection. However, when the diagnosis of MS is known, neurogenic bladder should be suspected as the possible cause. Clues to the presence of urinary tract infection include: burning or pain during urination (dysuria), increased frequency, urgency, incontinence, foul-smelling urine, pain in the lower back or abdomen, chills, and fever.

The presence of one or more of the preceding symptoms suggests neurogenic bladder but does not indicate the specific abnormality. This must be determined before treatment can begin, as dissimilar impairments can cause the same symptoms and require very different management. In general, bladder dysfunction in MS occurs when: (a) the bladder contracts poorly or excessively; (b) the urinary sphincter fails to relax; or (c) the actions of the muscle of the bladder wall and the sphincter are not properly coordinated.

These impairments of bladder function may differ, although the symptoms may be the same. Urgency, frequency, nocturia, and incontinence may be present in various kinds of bladder dysfunction. For this reason, it is crucial to identify the underlying defect. Without knowing the nature of the impairment, some measures to treat the symptoms may seem to be temporarily successful but may actually worsen the bladder's condition.

The two basic kinds of MS neurogenic bladder are:

Failure-to-store. Here the primary bladder muscle is overactive and signals an urge to urinate when less than 200 ml (less than a cup) of urine has collected in the bladder. This causes urgency, frequency, nocturia, and possibly incontinence.

Failure-to-empty. Here the primary bladder muscle may be weakened and not able to exert enough force to expel all urine from the bladder; the sphincter may be "tight" and hence not able to relax sufficiently to permit complete emptying (the urine left behind is called "residual urine").

The failure-to-store bladder does not allow the normal volume of urine to accumulate and is also referred to as a "small-capacity bladder." Accumulation of a small amount of urine creates the same need to urinate as that experienced by a person with normal bladder function when three to five times that quantity of urine has collected.

The failure-to-empty bladder may behave in a similar manner, with small amounts of urine being eliminated frequently. However, the retained urine (often not perceived by the individual) may continue to stretch the bladder. The result may be a "large-capacity bladder" which stretches the bladder muscle beyond recovery. At this point symptoms may actually diminish, as the damaged muscle ceases to signal the urge to void when the bladder is full. Urine may back up to the kidneys and cause substantial damage before the disorder is detected. Too often, awareness emerges when kidney involvement has created a crisis situation.

Some people with MS may present with a "mixed" type bladder with some elements of both failure-to-store and failure-to-empty syndromes. (A syndrome is a collection of symptoms and physical findings which fit within a known diagnostic classification.) These cases are also manageable, although a longer trial-and-error period may be needed to determine the most effective management.

DIAGNOSIS OF BLADDER DYSFUNCTION

In order to evaluate the individual situation, three steps are suggested: (a) detailed history of past and current bladder symptoms; (b) measurement of the amount of urine voided and the amount left behind (residual urine) after a concentrated effort to urinate voluntarily; and (c) laboratory testing to directly evaluate the ability of the bladder muscle to contract and the sphincter to relax.

Management is guided by these measures. Before the most effective treatment can be determined, a period of adjusting medications and techniques may be required.

Other tests are needed to periodically evaluate the MS patient's bladder function and the condition of his urinary tract. Understanding the purposes, procedures, and expected outcomes of these tests should allay fear and encourage the patient to actively participate in the sometimes lengthy process of bladder management.

History

The history of past and current bladder symptoms involves a dialogue between the patient and clinician about urinary problems which have occurred in the past, and the urinary disturbances which are present at the time of the evaluation. These might include the presence of urgency, frequency, nocturia, incontinence, infection, or other symptoms, as well as the type of diagnostic studies and procedures done in the past (such as prostate surgery). Former management measures, as well as bowel and sexual function, are discussed. This information will help to determine the best means for treating current problems by understanding the progression of urinary symptoms and the outcome of previous treatments.

Residual Urine

Residual urine determination gives the doctor important information about the present state of the patient's urinary system and his susceptibility to potentially serious complications. The "flushing" action of urine passing out of the body serves to expel waste, bacteria, and mineral deposits. Accumulated bacteria can multiply and lead to urinary tract infection, and retained mineral deposits may form urinary stones. The more urine left in the bladder after voiding, the greater is the risk of these complications.

The most useful way of determining residual urine is as follows:

1. When a strong desire to urinate is present, the patient attempts to empty the bladder using a commode (toilet chair with container) so that the voided amount may be measured.

2. After urinating, the nurse or physician inserts a thin, hollow tube (catheter) through the urinary opening into the bladder to drain the remaining urine. This procedure is quick, painless, and safe. It is helpful to know the amount voided as well as the amount of residual urine as the total amount reflects the bladder capacity—or amount of urine the bladder stores before it signals an urge to void. The combination of the voided volume plus the residual volume provides useful information that contributes to treatment decisions.

This test is utilized periodically to help determine how effective the treatment is. If the amount of residual urine decreases over a period of weeks or months, it indicates improved bladder function. Patients who are catheterizing themselves can provide this information to the physician or nurse, thereby actively participating in the management process.

Urodynamic Testing

In some individuals with bladder dysfunction, problems are identified by determining the pressure, or expulsive force, within the bladder and the capacity of the sphincter to contract or relax at appropriate times. This is called urodynamic testing.

The patient may be asked to drink a large amount of fluid prior to the test, depending on the technique used. The rectum should be empty, so laxatives or enemas may be advised for individuals prone to constipation. At the time of testing, a catheter is inserted through the urinary opening and left in place. A plug containing electrodes may be inserted into the rectum or a tiny needle with electrodes may be inserted directly into the urinary sphincter. Following this preparation, the patient rests comfortably while the bladder fills. He then may be called on to attempt bladder emptying, to cough, or to report changes in bladder sensation. The test is safe and painless and is essential in some situations in order to define what is wrong with the various mechanisms involved in voiding.

Other tests are performed depending on individual needs and are discussed below.

Cystoscopy

Cystoscopy is useful when an obstruction other than a tight sphincter is suspected (such as an enlarged prostate in older men). A thin tube with a light and magnifier is passed through the urinary opening so that the inside of the bladder can be examined visually.

Intravenous Pyelogram/Urogram

The entire urinary tract is visualized when an intravenous pyelogram or urogram, also called an IVP or an IVU, is undergone. This is a radiologic (x-ray) procedure. A special substance is injected into an arm vein; the material then circulates through the body and temporarily settles in the kidneys before it leaves the body in the urine. This allows the entire urinary system to be visualized via x-ray. "Intravenous" refers to injections into a vein; "pyelogram" is a kidney x-ray; and "urogram" describes the x-ray of the urinary system. Therefore IVU more accurately describes the test, although IVP is a better known term. Both terms refer to the same procedure. This evaluation should be performed about every 2 years for the individual with MS who experiences bladder symptoms. In this way, potentially serious complications may be identified at an early stage and corrected.

Urinalysis

The urine is tested to detect such abnormalities as the presence of bacteria, blood, or sugar. Results can be available within a few hours, and so the test is useful for screening purposes. If this "urinalysis" reveals abnormalities, more specific testing is needed. For example, the findings of many bacteria and a trace of blood suggest a urinary tract infection. However, the particular bacteria that are present and the drug that is most effective against them must be determined. This testing is called a urine culture (to grow the bacteria) and sensitivity tests (to determine the appropriate antibiotic to be used).

Urinary Culture and Sensitivity

A sterile urine specimen is required for culturing. It may be obtained by catheterization or by the "clean-catch" technique, which involves: (a) cleansing around the urinary opening; (b) passing a few drops of urine into the toilet to clear the urinary passage; (c) passing urine into a sterile container; and (d) keeping the specimen cold until delivered to the laboratory.

The urine is then placed on a culture medium in the laboratory and set aside for 48 hours to observe the absence or presence of bacterial growth. Should significant growth occur, the bacteria are identified and then tested against a series of antibiotics to determine which is most effective. The end result is identification of the antibiotic which can destroy that organism. When distressing symptoms accompany the infection, a broad-spectrum antibacterial agent may be given to the patient as soon as a urine culture is obtained. When the laboratory report is available several days later, the antibacterial agent may be continued if tests show it to be the correct one or changed if it does not adequately kill the bacteria that show up.

BLADDER MANAGEMENT

Failure to Store

The bladder fails to store urine when there is nervous system damage causing contractions of the bladder muscle which result in emptying before the bladder is filled to a normal capacity. The urge to urinate is then experienced when only a small amount of urine is present. The bladder is considered "hyperactive" and with a small capacity, as urine does not accumulate to the normal volume. The goal of management is to permit bladder filling to occur up to an adequate capacity before the urge to urinate is signaled.

This is accomplished by certain drugs. The specific drug must be prescribed by a physician. Side effects of the drugs used are the result of simultaneous slowing down of nervous system activity in other areas, notably the intestine and salivary glands. Therefore, constipation and dry mouth are likely occurrences. Constipation may be managed by measures described later in this chapter in the section dealing with bowel management. Dry mouth may be relieved by sucking on hard candy or rinsing the mouth with a commercial mouthwash. Blurred vision is another infrequent side effect which should be reported to the physician if it occurs. Most of these medications are administered cautiously to individuals with glaucoma, so the physician should be informed if glaucoma has been diagnosed or is suspected.

Failure to Empty

The failure-to-empty type of bladder dysfunction shows up as an inability to completely empty the bladder during voiding. This may be caused by bladder contractions of insufficient strength or duration to expel all of the urine in the bladder. A more common cause is incoordination of the bladder muscle and the sphincter. This means that when the bladder muscle provides an expulsive force to evacuate urine, the sphincter tightens instead of relaxing, thereby interfering with urination. In this situation the sphincter is referred to as "spastic," or "hyperactive."

Weak bladder muscle contractions may be strengthened by other drugs, such as bethanecol chloride. However, this is rarely indicated as beneficial effects are generally short-lived, and serious adverse effects can occur; moreover, a weakened bladder muscle is often seen together with a hyperactive sphincter. When these drugs are administered to a person with a hyperactive or spastic sphincter, the bladder contracts more forcefully but against a closed sphincter. This damages the bladder muscle and forms "pockets" where urine may collect; this, in turn, predisposes to urinary tract infection. Another danger is that urine can be forced to back up into the kidneys, thereby posing a serious threat to the patient's health.

In mild instances of failure to empty, an antispasticity drug (such as baclofen) may be effective in relaxing the sphincter, thereby helping to release the urine in the bladder. (See Chapter 5 for more detailed information about the various medications used for bladder management).

Bladder Training

Some affected individuals can train themselves to simulate normal voiding, keeping the following points in mind. Complete voiding is best performed on a toilet seat, as in this position pressure of internal organs does not cause pressure on the urethra and obstruct the outflow of urine. When the bladder is full and the desire to void is present, urine may flow. The flow may not last long enough and sometimes it may not occur. In that case, the bladder may be stimulated to contract by tapping the lower abdomen. If some urine comes out, the maneuver can be repeated as many times as is necessary until it produces no flow. Gently touching the urinary opening with a piece of toilet tissue may also release some urine. However, in most patients with the failure-to-empty disorder, intermittent catheterization is called for.

Intermittent Catheterization

Intermittent catheterization (IC) is a safe, easy, and effective means of emptying urine from the bladder. IC is performed by inserting a thin hollow tube (catheter) through the urinary opening for the purpose of eliminating all of the urine which has collected in the bladder. This is done several times a day to simulate normal voiding.

The primary goals of IC are to:

1. *Maintain the health of the urinary system.* This is accomplished by preventing recurrent urinary tract infections and secondary kidney (renal) impairment by: (a) *Eliminating residual urine.*

The inability to completely empty the bladder at each voiding provides a favorable medium for bacterial growth—similar to a stagnant pool of water—thereby fostering the development of urinary tract infections. Continuous or recurrent bladder infections may eventually involve the kidneys and create a serious health problem. (b) *Preventing bladder distention.* Filling the bladder beyond normal capacity reduces the bladder's inherent ability to fight off infection. The bladder muscle stretches, similar to a balloon that is filled with so much air that its walls become very thin. When this occurs with the bladder, its muscle fibers are stretched beyond their ability to function. Thus the weakened muscle cannot effectively expel urine, and large amounts of stagnant urine are retained. This process may be reversible if muscle fibers have not been destroyed by too much stretching. The sooner the process of bladder stretching is reversed, the more likely it is that recovery can occur. (c) *Preventing kidney damage caused by reflux.* Urine in a distended bladder may be forced back up the ureters toward the kidneys (reflux). Infected urine makes this particularly dangerous, as a kidney infection may result.

2. *Improve patient function.* Periodic complete emptying of the bladder often relieves complaints of urgency, frequency, nocturia, and incontinence, especially when combined with appropriate medication. The length of time between urinating should be increased and "accidents" hopefully eliminated.

3. *Restore bladder function.* Periodic emptying of the distended bladder frequently promotes the return of bladder muscle strength. Following 3 to 4 months of IC, bladder function may approach normal, eliminating the need for continuing IC. Although restoration of function is not possible for everyone, it is considered a goal during the evaluation and management process.

Technique

Although IC is generally considered valuable, various techniques are used. Most health professionals who teach IC to patients in the community advise some form of the "clean" technique. This means that strict sterile practices (such as the use of sterile gloves) are not required. The rationale is that the bladder has a natural tendency to resist infection so long as it is emptied periodically. The basic guidelines for the patient performing IC are as follows:

1. Wash the hands.
2. Attempt to urinate.
3. Clean around the urinary opening.
4. Insert a lubricated catheter and drain the urine.
5. Remove the catheter and either: (a) discard the catheter; (b) wash and store it; or (c) wash, boil, and store it.
6. Periodically measure the amount urinated and the residual urine, keeping a dated record of these numbers. Voided and residual amounts provide an ongoing assessment of bladder function and will help the physician determine when IC can be decreased or discontinued.

For those patients who require IC several times a day, the technique should be designed to fit comfortably into the daily routine. When IC is performed on a regular basis, relief of symptoms encourages continuation of the procedure. For men, the urinary opening is visible, and the technique is easily mastered by those with the ability to use their hands. Women, however, have the urethral opening (meatus) located outside of direct vision. This situation is approached in the same manner as learning to insert a tampon. A mirror should be used to identify the meatus. During practice sessions, inserting a tampon into the vagina is helpful; with the vagina blocked, only one opening is left for inserting the catheter (Fig. 2). Continued use of a mirror needlessly complicates the technique.

IC may need to be performed by someone other than the patient when severe motor or sensory disability interferes with self-insertion. A family member or home attendant may be taught to perform this function. IC is far more preferable to a catheter that is left in the bladder, as the latter has the greater risk of complications.

Additional applications of IC should be noted. Women who experience incontinence during sexual intercourse can perform IC prior to sexual activity. Also those who utilize IC on a regular basis may alter their schedule when desired (such as prior to a shopping ex-

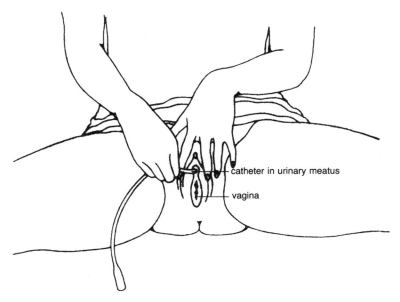

FIG. 2. Technique of female self catheterization.

pedition). This flexibility enhances the person's control over his/her bladder function.

Mixed Neurogenic Bladder

The mixed neurogenic bladder has features of both the failure-to-store and failure-to-empty disorders. The sphincter is tight and does not allow the bladder to empty completely. However, even when the patient can empty his/her bladder (usually because IC is done), the hyperactive bladder signals the urge to urinate when only a small amount of urine has collected. Medication is needed to relax the bladder and allow a normal amount of urine to collect. The bladder can then be emptied by conveniently scheduled IC.

INDWELLING CATHETERS

There are certain situations when it is best to use a catheter which remains inside the bladder. The usual type of this "indwelling catheter" is called a "Foley catheter." This is a thin, hollow tube that is inserted into the bladder and connected to an external drainage bag. The catheter is kept in the bladder by a small balloon that is inflated after insertion. The catheter is easily removed by deflating this balloon through an external valve.

The conditions which might indicate a need for temporary use of an indwelling catheter are as follows:

1. A person whose bladder has been excessively stretched by urinary retention for several months may benefit from a few weeks of this type of urinary drainage. Although IC is preferred, it is not always possible due to the person's severe disability and the absence of someone else to carry out the procedure on a regular basis. The expectation is that the bladder muscle may regain some degree of normal function by relieving the pressure and stretching caused by urinary retention.

2. When someone other than the MS person performs IC, and it is necessary for this individual to be absent for several days or more, a Foley catheter may have to be used.

3. If pressure sores develop on the buttocks or other areas close to the urinary opening, a Foley catheter may be needed to eliminate urinary incontinence, a factor which impedes healing of the pressure sores.

4. Following surgical procedures that involve the urinary or reproductive systems or after difficult childbirth, indwelling catheterization may be needed until the swelling of surrounding tissues subsides and urinary flow may resume unobstructed.

5. Certain social or travel situations may present obstacles to urination or to IC. Important social functions (such as weddings) may not be held in places with accessible toilets. This is also usually true with various travel modes as well (bus, train, airplane). A Foley catheter may be a comfortable way of overcoming such barriers to pleasurable experiences. Ideally, a catheter in these situations should not be left in for more than 24 hours. Beyond this time, bacterial growth in the bladder is almost inevitable and increases the risk of bladder infection.

Some of the situations which necessitate long-term indwelling catheterization include the following:

1. Severe disability which precludes self-catheterization or the unavailability of another individual who can perform IC on a regular basis.

2. Female incontinence resistant to all other efforts at control.

3. In the case of occasional incontinence in women who are at great risk from their susceptibility to skin ulceration.

4. Females who have had several occurrences of pressure sores and need to avoid any possibility of urinary incontinence.

5. Obese women who are unable to stand and cannot transfer, alone or assisted, to a toilet or commode because of excessive body weight.

6. Females who are prevented by emotional or intellectual disturbances from participating in alternate measures of bladder management.

Indwelling catheterization is prescribed more often for women than men. This is because of sex-related anatomical differences rather than "sex discrimination." The penis provides a convenient appendage for attachment of an external drainage device. This is not possible for females due to the location of their urinary opening.

Care of Indwelling Catheters

The indwelling catheter can be managed at home with minimal effort. It is inserted using sterile technique and is changed every 4 to 6 weeks, or more frequently if blockage occurs. The community's visiting nurse association will generally provide this service when it is requested by a physician. The catheter insertion kit should be obtained prior to the nurse's visit. Other supplies needed are: a leg bag, a night bag, betadine solution, sterile gauze or cotton balls, alcohol, an irrigation set, saline solution, and vinegar.

Daily care consists of cleaning around the catheter insertion site with sterile cotton or gauze soaked with betadine solution in the morning and the evening. An individual with an indwelling catheter needs to drink an adequate or even an excessive amount of fluids— 2 to 3 quarts a day. Fluids should be selected which promote urinary acidity, thereby deterring bacterial growth. This excludes such juices as orange, grapefruit, and tomato, while encouraging intake of cranberry, apple, apricot, and prune juices. Vitamin C, at a dose of 1,000 mg four times a day, is also recommended for this purpose. A urinary antiseptic is also advised but must be prescribed by a physician.

When changing from the leg bag worn during the day to a night bag, connecting pieces should be wiped with alcohol to impede the entrance of bacteria. Collection bags (leg and night) can be rinsed with warm water, then deodorized by a mixture of warm water and vinegar left soaking in the bag for a few hours.

Leakage of urine around the catheter tube or expulsion of the catheter has several possible causes, and these must be systematically examined:

1. *Obstructed catheter drainage.* The small drainage holes of the catheter may become blocked by mucus or sediment, requiring irrigation to clear the passageway. The irrigation set and saline are utilized for this purpose. The procedure can be carried out by the visiting nurse or by an individual in the household instructed in the proper technique.

2. *Adequate fluid intake.* If insufficient fluid is drunk, the urine will be concentrated and may serve as an irritant to the bladder, causing vigorous contractions which force urine out around the drainage tube. It is essential that fluid intake be at least 2 to 3 quarts a day.

3. *Urinary tract infection.* Infected urine may act as an irritant, stimulating bladder contractions. If this occurs, a urine specimen must be checked in the laboratory for the presence of bacteria: a culture and sensitivity test should be done.

4. *Bladder muscle spasms.* The neurogenic bladder may have uninhibited spasms that intermittently force urine out around the catheter. This may be controlled by a medication such as propantheline bromide.

5. *Oversized catheter or retaining balloon.* A catheter or retaining balloon which is too large is irritating and causes inflammation. An oversized catheter or balloon is sometimes unfortunately used as a "plug" to control leakage without exploring possible causes.

Other long-term problems may result when an oversized catheter is used inappropriately.

SURGICAL PROCEDURES

There are no surgical procedures that can return the bladder to normal functioning. The primary goals of therapy are to promote bladder emptying, relieve symptoms, and subsequently reduce debilitating, possibly life-threatening complications. A few surgical procedures can help achieve these goals under special circumstances. The most common are suprapubic cystostomy, vesicostomy, sphincterotomy, and transurethral resection.

Cystostomy

Cystostomy is a surgically created opening into the urinary bladder through the lower abdomen. A catheter is inserted through the new opening and connected by plastic tubing to a collection device (leg bag/night bag). Urine flows through the catheter rather than through the natural urinary opening. The operation is not a major procedure and requires the patient to be in a hospital for only a few days.

The reasons for using this approach are similar to those calling for the use of a permanent indwelling catheter. Moreover, it is easily taken care of—in a fashion similar to that for the urethral catheter—and injuries to the urethra may be avoided. Cystostomy is only occasionally necessary. An additional measure is use of a gauze pad cut to surround the cystostomy tube and held in place with hypoallergenic tape.

Continent Vesicostomy

Continent vesicostomy, which is potentially helpful to only a small number of individuals, also involves surgical creation of a new outlet for urinary drainage in the lower abdomen. However, a catheter is not left in the bladder with this procedure. Instead, intermittent catheterization through the small abdominal opening is employed for periodic urinary drainage. There are special considerations for choosing this procedure. These include: (a) a bladder with a normal to large capacity so that drainage may be scheduled four to six times a day; (b) an inability of the patient to self-catheterize using the natural urinary opening and the unavailability of a suitable person to regularly catheterize the patient; (c) longstanding urinary retention that is unresponsive to more conservative management and which is not likely to clear spontaneously.

This procedure is recommended only after careful consideration of many physical/psychological/social factors. Several weeks must be set aside for the procedure, with a brief hospitalization for surgery followed by a postoperative period of "cystostomy" type urinary drainage. When it is indicated, however, continent vesicostomy provides a safe and generally acceptable means of bladder management.

Sphincterotomy

In the severely spastic male who cannot empty his bladder despite all efforts, the sphincter can be enlarged surgically. An inability to control urination results, but it can be managed in males by an external collecting device. Females are not candidates for the procedure because urinary drainage cannot be managed without the danger of skin breakdown.

Transurethral Resection

When a patient has had an indwelling catheter for a long time and the pressure of the balloon of the Foley catheter has irritated the bladder neck (the area where the bladder connects with the urethra), the tissues may become thickened and obstruct the flow of urine when the catheter is removed. In that case, the excess tissue of the bladder neck is removed, which then allows the urine to flow freely. The procedure is required only rarely and most often in males.

There are other procedures that may be advocated, but most of them are indicated only rarely and should be undertaken with careful consideration.

BOWEL MANAGEMENT

Most people with MS gave little thought to bowel function before the onset of their illness. Many continue without bowel dysfunction throughout the course of the disease. However, for those who are currently having bowel problems, or who have an interest in understanding the causes and management of bowel dysfunction in MS, this section is relevant.

The most common bowel complaint of the person with MS is constipation. There are several factors which cause or contribute to this problem. However, regardless of the underlying cause or causes, management measures are the same. Loss of bowel control (bowel incontinence) is an infrequent but very disturbing occurrence in MS.

Constipation

Constipation is defined as a condition in which bowel movements are infrequent or incomplete. "Infrequent" bowel movement is defined as occurring less often than every 3 days. "Incomplete" refers to part or most of the stool being retained in the rectum or lower intestine following attempts to have a bowel movement (defecate). Perception as to what is normal needs to be examined in light of this. It is not necessary to have a daily bowel movement, but defecation once a week or less often is outside the acceptable range. Stool which is increasingly retained in the lower digestive tract tends to stretch the bowel, thereby weakening its ability to move waste out of the body. Also, the longer the stool is retained in the intestine, the more of its water content is withdrawn by the body. This creates a dry, hardened stool which is increasingly difficult to evacuate.

In addition to the obvious effects of constipation, more subtle events also occur. Stool retained in the rectum may cause pressure on parts of the urinary system, thereby increasing bladder disturbance. Stretching of the rectum by retained stool sends messages to the spinal cord, which further disturbs bladder function and adversely affects walking because of increased spasticity. This information is important, as many people view constipation as a localized annoyance. Understanding this pattern enhances awareness of the benefits of an effective bowel program for individuals with MS.

Constipation may also directly result from MS involvement of that portion of the nervous system that controls bowel function. This produces a "sluggish bowel," which moves waste slowly through the digestive system. As with incomplete emptying, the body then absorbs a greater amount of water from the stool (feces), leaving hardened stool which is difficult to pass. Another indirect MS influence on bowel movements is weakened abdominal muscles. This makes it difficult to "bear down" strongly enough to create sufficient pressure within the abdomen for easy evacuation of stool. The result is constipation.

Decreased physical activity due to impaired walking or easy fatigability is a common secondary cause of sluggish bowel activity. Constipation also results when the amount of fluid a person drinks is voluntarily reduced. This most often happens when urinary complaints, such as urgency, frequency, and loss of control (incontinence), are present. In this situation, fluid restriction is intended to minimize urinary problems, although constipation is a predictable outcome. Another contributing factor is postponement of defecation, once awareness of a full rectum is experienced. Certain types of drugs are also known to promote constipation. These include pain relievers containing narcotics (such as codeine), some medications used to treat urinary symptoms, and antacids containing aluminum. Chronic harsh laxative use eventually increases constipation. As the laxative effect wears off, there is a "rebound" reaction of the bowel to a more sluggish state than prior to the laxative use.

Management is discussed here by first outlining general measures to promote good bowel function. This is followed by specific measures, listed according to the order in which they should be utilized. An adequate trial should be attempted at each level. An important point is that any trial of bowel management requires several weeks before effectiveness can be evaluated, as a gradual modification of the digestive rhythm is involved.

General Measures to Promote Good Bowel Function

1. Adequate fluid intake of at least 2 quarts a day. Include coffee, juice, or whatever fluids are desired.
2. Daily intake of fiber (such as bran cereal) to provide water-retaining bulk in the stool. This stimulates movement of the stool

toward the rectum (see *Fiber Diet Planner*, a booklet available free from Kellogg's for a detailed diet).

3. Regular physical activity including exercise. This may range from swimming to wheelchair exercises. Whatever physical activity is reasonable for the individual will be helpful.

4. Evacuation at the same time of day. The best time to attempt defecation is one-half hour after mealtime when the emptying reflex (gastrocolic reflex) is strongest.

Measures to Manage Resistant Constipation

1. All of the above.

2. Stool softeners (such as Colace) daily.

3. Bulk supplements (natural fiber supplements), such as Metamucil, daily.

4. Mild oral laxatives, such as milk of magnesia, on alternate nights or nightly if needed.

5. Glycerin suppository one-half hour prior to planned evacuation. This may be needed for several weeks during the period of regulating the bowel, or it may be used indefinitely.

6. Bisocodyl (Dulcolax) suppositories when glycerin suppositories have proved ineffective.

7. Fleet enema at the time of planned evacuation periodically when usual measures have been ineffective, or on a regular basis if absolutely necessary. This measure is used in conjunction with stool softeners, bulk supplements, and mild oral laxatives.

Measures to Manage Severe and Longstanding Constipation in the Severely Disabled Person

1. An adequate trial of all the above measures.

2. Medical evaluation to check out possible contributing factors other than MS.

3. Tap water enema every 2 to 3 days in conjunction with previously mentioned fluid intake, dietary fiber, stool softeners, laxatives, and/or suppositories as indicated by the benefit observed.

The tap water enema may also be used periodically when routinely practiced measures are ineffective.

4. Manual removal of hardened feces in the rectum by inserting the index and middle fingers into the rectum (rubber glove and lubricant required). This is an infrequently needed technique for the severely debilitated person who is normally regulated by other measures.

An additional technique for individuals who find it difficult to completely empty the rectum is digital stimulation of the anal opening. Insertion of the index finger (covered with a latex "finger cot") through the anal sphincter, with gentle rotation of the finger, may be sufficient to stimulate rectal emptying. The technique should be used only periodically as chronic anal stretching may cause damage to the anal sphincter. It is also important to note the impact of varying dietary habits on bowel function. Individuals differ in their response to specific foods, and this needs to be considered when determining an overall bowel program.

Bowel Incontinence

Total loss of bowel control is a very rare occurrence in MS, but it does affect some severely disabled individuals. Episodic loss of bowel control, however, can occur when there is only minimal MS impairment. This is a very distressing and difficult problem to resolve.

Bowel incontinence occurs: (a) when there is loose stool and intestinal upset, such as when the patient has flu; (b) when MS affects the intestine or anal sphincter; and (c) occasionally when non-MS-related bowel problems are present. Therefore, when a fair trial of regulatory measures is unsuccessful or when bowel incontinence persists beyond an acute flu-type illness, a gastroenterologist (a doctor specializing in gastrointestinal disorders) should be consulted. Non-MS bowel problems may be then identified and treated with a greater degree of success.

Loose stool present during episodes of incontinence may be responsible for the bowel accidents, as the anal sphincter cannot easily contain liquid. Loose stool may result from common viral or flu-type syndromes, and in those instances the problem will solve itself. Dietary factors may be the cause for some individuals, and a test elimination of substances which irritate the gut (such as spicy food, coffee, alcohol, and cigarettes) may be effective. Loose stool can also be passed around a blockage of hardened feces in the lower intestine or rectum. This blockage is called impaction and requires aggressive efforts, including an oil retention enema or tap water enema, for correction. Establishment of an effective bowel program which is followed faithfully usually prevents recurrence of this problem.

MS involvement that is responsible for occasional, or in some severely disabled persons frequent, loss of bowel control can be caused by sensory loss in the rectum. Rectal filling may be partially or totally unperceived, allowing the rectum to stretch beyond the usual capacity. An unexpected, involuntary relaxation of the anal sphincter may occur, resulting in bowel incontinence. The most effective way (currently known) to combat this problem is to establish a regular bowel program and stay with it. When the bowel is trained to empty at regular intervals, accidents are less likely.

In these cases the measures for bowel regulation will include those used to manage constipation. Adequate fluid intake, fiber in the diet, exercise, and possibly a suppository to stimulate a bowel movement at the scheduled time exemplifies a possible program. An important point is that a daily bowel movement is not necessary—the regularity of the time interval (such as every other day) and the time of day (such as always after breakfast) are the important time factors.

During the period of bowel training (which may be several weeks or months) while incontinence is a concern, a few suggestions may be helpful. It is very important to be alert to signals that suggest the need to defecate about 30 minutes after meals. A reflex that encourages bowel emptying (gastrocolic reflex) occurs at this time, suggesting that this is a prime time for an accident if one is likely to occur. Also, coffee and other hot liquids may stimulate a rapid response from the digestive system and a precipitous urge to defecate. For these individuals who find bowel incontinence a frequent problem, protective underpants are recommended (such as Attends). An absorbent lining helps protect the skin, and a plastic outer shield inhibits release of odor and shields clothing from being soiled.

Some innovative ways to control bowel incontinence are being explored. The most notable is biofeedback. This technique involves sensitizing the individual to subtle signals of rectal filling to compensate for diminished normal mechanisms. Although this technique is still in the exploratory stage, it exemplifies the possibilities for management which may be available in the near future.

Bowel management is often a tedious, frustrating experience. Trial and error is usually involved, and success may be measured by small accomplishments at infrequent intervals. However, persistence is usually rewarded with some sense of control over bowel function and a subsequent release from the continuing worry over the effects of bowel dysfunction.

SUMMARY

Problems with urination and bowel function occur in the majority of individuals with MS at some time during the course of the disease. Symptoms in these areas frequently remit and should not be viewed as a permanent disability. Successful management is possible in most cases. Symptoms can be relieved, complications prevented, and irreversible damage to the urinary tract and bowel avoided. However, the MS person must openly communicate the specific symptoms to the physician and be aggressive in seeking the necessary help.

11

Sexuality

Rosalind Kalb, Nicholas LaRocca, and Seymour R. Kaplan

Sexuality is an important part of life and of relating to others. It plays a significant role in determining how a person feels about him- or herself. The average person between the ages of 20 and 50 today faces a variety of complex pressures in relation to sex. Most people bring from childhood certain taboos or inhibitions which make it difficult to discuss sexual problems or feelings. At the same time, the current social/sexual milieu in our culture places a heavy emphasis on sexual expression, openness, and experimentation.

This apparent contradiction has both negative and positive implications for the disabled person. On the one hand, an MS patient confronted with a variety of sexual problems may have no one (perhaps not even a spouse) with whom he can comfortably talk about sexual matters. The individual may not even be comfortable thinking about these problems. This difficulty is then compounded by the current emphasis on sexuality and freedom of sexual expression. The individual is left feeling inadequate and frustrated, with no place to turn for help. From a more positive perspective, however, the current emphasis on sexual freedom may make it easier for the individual with sexual problems to consider varied or alternative modes of sexual expression.

Sexual intercourse in the more traditional man-on-top position is no longer the only "acceptable" means of expressing one's sexuality. Many individuals, with or without disability, are feeling freer to engage in oral or anal sex, masturbatory activities with or without a partner, or other sexual activities which they find satisfying and pleasurable. The current popular literature is filled with sexual how-to books which describe varied ways of giving and receiving sexual pleasure and satisfaction before, during, or apart from intercourse.

MS is a complex and difficult disease which requires an ongoing, open relationship between the person with the disease and his or her sexual partner. The material presented here will hopefully serve as a useful tool in this dialogue rather than as a substitute for it. All too frequently, sexual difficulties are ignored or denied because neither partner feels comfortable acknowledging or discussing them.

Sexual problems also need to be discussed with a physician or other knowledgeable and supportive health care professional. Such individuals may prove to be valuable resources in the ongoing coping process. Unfortunately, physicians often ignore sexual problems or hesitate to question their patients about this sensitive issue. The MS person may need to take the initiative in discussing sexual problems with the doctor. The joint efforts of patient, partner, and physician need to be directed toward accomplishing the successful and satisfying management of whatever sexual problems may develop.

NORMAL SEXUAL FUNCTIONING

Sexual response occurs in two separate phases which are similar in both men and women. The first phase involves vasocongestion. In males, blood is carried to, and trapped within, special parts of the penis, causing it to become erect. Similarly in the female, swelling occurs in the blood vessels of the labia and tissues of the vagina resulting in vaginal lubrication and expansion of the vaginal walls. This initial arousal phase can occur in response to two types of stimulation: physical contact including kissing and caressing, and erotic thoughts or mental images. Arousal in response to mental images is said to be psychogenic in origin and is controlled by the higher brain center.

Orgasm is the second phase of sexual response. In males, orgasm consists of two phases, emission and ejaculation. Emission is the reflex contraction of the internal reproductive organs, experienced by men as the sensation of imminent ejaculation. Emission is followed almost immediately by ejaculation, a series of contractions of the muscles at the base of the penis. In contrast, the female orgasm involves only one process consisting of a similar series of muscle contractions.

Following orgasm males experience a refractory period of variable length during which sexual arousal is reduced and they are unable to reach another orgasm. Females, however, have no such refractory period. They can usually have repeated orgasms without a reduction in arousal level.

SEXUAL DIFFICULTIES RELATED TO MS

Sexual functioning of persons with MS may be profoundly influenced by the physical and emotional effects of the disease. Lilius surveyed 302 people with MS and found that 91% of the men and 77% of the women reported a change in their sexual lives. Only 20% of the men in their survey reported an adequate erection. Women mentioned inability to achieve orgasm (33%), loss of libido (27%), and spasticity interfering with sex (12%) as their chief difficulties. Clearly, sexual functioning represents an area of concern for people with MS. Although these statistics may appear distressing, two important points should be kept in mind: First, people with MS are not alone in experiencing sexual problems. In any typical "happily married" sample of individuals, a large percentage report sexual problems, many of which are similar to some of the difficulties related to MS. Second, "successful" sex does not have to be defined as having an erection, having intercourse, or having an orgasm. The satisfaction achieved in sexual contact comes from three major sources: pleasurable physical sensations, affectionate closeness with another person, and the gratifying feeling of performing successfully and giving pleasure. The potential problems caused by MS can, of course, interfere with any one or all of these sources of satisfaction at one time or another.

The aim here is to demonstrate how people can learn to achieve satisfaction in varying ways when and if the need arises and perhaps even to redefine for themselves what feels good or is sexually satisfying. The remainder of this chapter points out the difficulties most frequently reported by individuals with MS. The problems fall into four major areas: those resulting from the neurophysiological changes of MS, those caused by possible physical changes, psychological conflicts and pressures related to disability, and problems resulting from social pressures and attitudes.

Although it is useful for individuals with MS and their sexual partners to understand the various causes of their sexual problems, it may be even more useful and satisfying to learn how others have successfully tackled these problems.

Sexual Difficulties Related to the Neurophysiological Changes of MS

Because MS may affect many parts of the central nervous system, almost any part of the sexual response may be affected. MS may impair a person's ability to become sexually aroused, resulting in unsatisfactory penile erection or vaginal lubrication. However, even in those individuals where this arousal response is impaired, a reflex response may remain. For example, the person might be unable to achieve erection via sexual thoughts but respond with a reflex erection when the penis is stroked. Other individuals experience the opposite phenomenon. The perineal (genital area) reflex may be lost, but the person can still become sexually aroused in response to visual or emotional stimulation.

Sensations in the genital area may be totally or partially lost due to MS. When the sensations are only partly lost, stimulation that at one time felt good may begin to feel irritating or even painful. These sensory changes can interfere with a person's ability to feel pleasurable sensations, and this in turn can interfere with the ability to ejaculate or have an orgasm. Problems in the autonomic nervous system—the system which controls automatic, nonvoluntary bodily actions (such as digestion) or reactions—can also cause problems with erection or vaginal lubrication. If MS has affected the "higher" brain centers—those involved in thoughts and emotions—there may be changes in sexual desire and arousal. Other changes in these same centers may interfere with a person's ability to communicate clearly with the sexual partner.

It is clear from these examples that MS can produce a variety of central nervous system changes which directly affect the sexual response. Like other MS symptoms caused by changes in the central nervous system, these neurologically based changes in sexual feelings have no absolute "cure." However, it is often possible to circumvent these problems through some combination of creativity, flexibility, and possible sexual aids and/or prosthetic devices.

The neurologically caused erectile and ejaculatory difficulties experienced by many men with MS generally do not remit, although their frequency or regularity of occurrence differs from one individual to another. The first step in the management of these difficulties is a frank discussion with a physician or other knowledgeable health professional. This individual can help the person with MS determine to what extent the difficulties are a result of neurological impairment and what role psychological factors (such as performance anxiety or depression) may be playing. The man with MS can help in this effort by becoming familiar with his own body and its functioning. The following are questions he needs to answer for himself: "Am I able to achieve and maintain an erection by any means, either during intercourse or through masturbation?" "Do I ever awaken in the night or early morning with an erection?" If the answer to either of these questions is "yes," neurological impairment is probably not total. This means that the person can sometimes achieve and maintain an erection by direct stimulation of the penis. If the answer to the questions is "no," neurological impairment is likely to be more extensive and the problems may be more permanent. An additional question the person needs to ask himself is: "Am I experiencing bowel or bladder difficulties, such as feelings of urgency, frequency of urination, or incontinence?" In MS, sexual problems caused by neurological changes are frequently accompanied by bowel and bladder problems.

The second step in the management of erectile problems involves specific techniques. In those individuals who can achieve reflex erections by stroking the penis, intercourse is possible, though probably without ejaculation. This can be a satisfying solution for those men who can derive sexual pleasure primarily from pleasing their partner. If a man is able to have an erection or feels physically aroused only infrequently, it will be important for him to learn how to identify those times and take advantage of them. Here again, awareness of his own body and the ability to share this with his partner is necessary.

Men should be aware that orgasm may occur without visible ejaculation. This is caused by *retrograde ejaculation*, where the semen is ejaculated back into the bladder. This may be alarming to the person but is *not harmful*. Retrograde ejaculation does prevent conception, however, and couples who wish to have children should discuss this problem with a urologist or a fertility specialist.

Penile prostheses are a possible alternative for men with chronic erectile problems who strongly wish to engage in intercourse. Currently there are three main types of prosthesis, each with its own advantages and disadvantages. The *noninflatable rod type* prosthesis consists of two sponge-filled rods that are surgically inserted into the shaft of the penis. These rods create a permanent semierection. The advantages of this prosthesis include a relatively simple and inexpensive surgical procedure that requires less than a week of hospitalization and is associated with few complications. With the rod-type device, however, the penis is constantly semierect and therefore difficult to conceal. Also, the penis is smaller than it is with an inflatable device (see below), and problems can occur which require reimplantation.

The newest type of prosthetic device is a *flexible* version of the rod type implant. A flexible, silver rod coated with soft plastic is implanted into the penile shaft. The penis remains in a constant semierect state but can be bent upward at the angle of an erect penis or downward at the nonerect angle for easier concealment.

The *inflatable type* prosthesis has more advantages and disadvantages than the rod type implants. The erection process with this device simulates the normal process and therefore allows greater psychological satisfaction. The erect penis is larger than it is with the rod device and has a normal nonerect appearance when not inflated. The device does not interfere with urinary function. This prosthesis, however, is relatively expensive and requires more extensive and costly surgery. More than a week of hospitalization is required, and the postoperative recovery period is significantly longer. There are also several possible complications: inflammation of the glans penis, tightness of the foreskin, and problems with the silicone tubing that can require reimplantation. In addition, the inflatable prothesis is somewhat difficult to operate. The small "pump" which inflates the device is implanted within the scrotum and can be difficult to locate. Newer models of the inflatable prosthesis have sought to overcome many of these problems, making this a more attractive solution than it had been.

Women who experience difficulties becoming aroused or reaching orgasm due to neurological changes are also encouraged to talk problems over with a knowledgeable health care professional and to become as familiar as possible with their own bodies. If and when sexual feelings and sensations change, each woman can then learn for herself and convey to her partner what is and is not pleasurable to her. Such changes in women, even if temporary, can nevertheless be frustrating and uncomfortable, making open communication with the partner essential.

Women who are experiencing decreased vaginal lubrication should use a sterile, water-soluble jelly such as K-Y. Vaseline should never be used because it is not water-soluble, and may cause severe urinary tract infection.

Painful genital sensations in either men or women are best relieved by the same medications used for other sensory problems of MS such as trigeminal neuralgia (facial pain) or assorted paresthesias (sensations of burning, tingling, crawling, or constriction). Tegretol (carbamazepine) is the drug of choice for these problems, with Dilantin (diphenylhydantoin) as a second choice when Tegretol is not effective. If disturbing or painful genital sensations have replaced pleasurable ones, or pleasurable sensations are lost because of numbness or anesthesia in the genital area, individuals can learn to identify other areas of their bodies which respond sexually. This process occurs through experimentation and frank discussion with the sexual partner. Individuals and couples who are forced to be innovative often "discover" parts of their bodies and sexual techniques they had never before thought of or tried. Oral and manual stimulation of different parts of the body can often be a very satisfying alternative to or sometime substitute for intercourse. If an individual or a couple can no longer enjoy intercourse as they once did either because of erectile problems, ejaculatory/orgasmic difficulties, or painful genital sensations, this does *not* mean it is no longer possible to feel close and give and receive pleasure.

For some people masturbation is an acceptable and satisfying alternative to intercourse. If a person is experiencing uncomfortable genital sensations or difficulty becoming sexually aroused, s/he may discover that s/he can attain sexual satisfaction more easily and comfortably through self-stimulation than by trying to describe to a partner just what does or does not feel good. Masturbation can be a "successful," intimate, shared experience with a partner or a satisfying and relaxing experience when done alone.

Honest discussion of sexual feelings and activities is heartily encouraged. Some individuals find it difficult to talk about sexual topics, such as anatomy, variations of the sex act, or what feels good. Shared reading material can often be a very helpful introduction to frank discussion. Books or pamphlets can provide the vocabulary and visual images which many people may be too inhibited to use on their own.

Sexual Difficulties Relating to Physical Changes

Bodily changes which do not directly affect the sexual response can, however, interfere with a satisfactory sexual life. Fatigue may affect a person's level of sexual interest and make it difficult to initiate or carry on sexual activity. Individuals with MS frequently report that by evening, when the sexual partner is home and available for sex, they are just too tired to enjoy it. The primary solution to the problem of fatigue is to conserve energy whenever possible. Use of a motorized wheelchair or cart (such as an Amigo or Portascoot) can relieve fatigue. Allowing for frequent rest periods during the course of the day is also beneficial. Making use of morning time for sexual activity when most individuals with MS feel strongest, can maximize energy and interest levels. In addition, medication (such as Cylert, a central nervous system stimulant which is not an amphetamine and has few side effects) is sometimes helpful in the relief of lassitude and fatigue.

It is also helpful to remember that sexual activity is not a contest or an athletic marathon. It can be a time of closeness, holding, sharing, and talking. If physical activity is possible and feels good, it is there to be enjoyed; otherwise partners can experiment with other ways of loving and giving and feeling pleasure.

Weakness, pain, stiffness, spasticity, or contractures can make certain movements or positions difficult to achieve. At times it becomes impossible to find a comfortable position for satisfying sexual activities. Tremors or incoordination may make even the simplest or gentlest movements impossible or awkward. Medications and surgical procedures for these problems are discussed in Chapter 7.

In general, sexual interaction may be complicated by concerns about a variety of possible physical problems, including loss of bowel or bladder control, personal hygiene, pain, pressure sores, or urinary tract infections. Each partner may silently wonder to what extent the other harbors such concerns. The MS individual may feel fragile, uncertain, or even afraid of sexual contact. These feelings are easily transmitted to a partner who, in turn, holds back and feels anxious and inhibited. Here again, the ability to share these feelings with a partner leads to greater relaxation and intimacy. In fact, the intimacy and trust that can be achieved through greater openness can replace some of what might be lost in reduced sexual activity.

Couples frequently report that their sexual lives have become so encumbered that any chance at sexual spontaneity is lost. For a couple in which one partner is severely disabled, so much planning and arranging is required for sexual activity that it becomes difficult to feel relaxed, uninhibited, or spontaneous. Couples can learn to be creative in dealing with this particular kind of problem. First, to the extent that it is possible, nursing activities should be carried out by someone other than a family member so that the disabled partner can retain the role and feelings of being a partner rather than a patient. It is also important that a couple's bedroom not be turned into a sickroom. The reality in our culture is that illness and sexuality are not usually thought of together. It is easier to have sexual feelings when not surrounded by nursing equipment. Second, preparation for sexual activity can always be accompanied by intimate conversation, relaxing music, even a little wine if bladder control is not a problem. The preparation for sex becomes part of the sexual activity rather than a tiresome preamble. Third, it is extremely important for men and women with MS to continue to try to look and feel as attractive as they possibly can. The need for a catheter or a wheelchair should in no way lessen a person's need to be clean, stylish, and neat. A person who feels attractive will be more confident and more relaxed about sex and therefore more sexually attractive to his or her partner.

Loss of bladder or bowel control, or the use of a urinary catheter, can cause considerable inconvenience and anxiety to sexual partners. There is a two-step process involved in coping with this problem. First, it is necessary for people with MS to learn about bladder and bowel problems and their management. The medical and mechanical aspects of these symptoms are discussed fully in Chapter 10.

Bladder symptoms such as urgency and frequency of urination and incontinence are often relieved by some combination of the following: a modified fluid intake (especially during the few hours before going to bed), scheduling regular bowel movements, medication, and intermittent catheterization. Individuals must experiment, in collaboration with their doctor, until the most satisfactory solution is found. Although this process may take time and patience, successful bladder management is essential for good health and peace of mind, both of which are important ingredients in a satisfactory sex life. Urinary tract infections can result when the bladder is not properly managed. These infections are uncomfortable and require prompt medical attention, but they are *not* transmitted to a sexual partner.

Because of the degree of constipation experienced by most people with MS, bowel incontinence during sex is less likely to occur. In general, bowel incontinence is most effectively prevented with a carefully managed regimen of bowel evacuation several times weekly.

The bowel management regimen can include modifications in diet, stool softeners, mild laxatives, suppositories, and in the case of long-term intractable problems, enemas. The use of any of these measures should be reviewed with a physician.

The second step in bowel and bladder management is more difficult to achieve, for it involves ongoing openness and flexibility between sexual partners. Both partners need to be able to express their honest feelings about these problems. The feelings may include anxiety, anger, disgust, or inhibition of sexual arousal. Any and all of these emotional responses are normal, and couples need to be able to share them without feeling guilty. Being able to talk freely about these feelings will help to reduce their intensity. This will enable the partners to support each other more easily through any necessary changes or adjustments in their sex life.

Psychological Conflicts

Individuals coping with MS frequently experience marked changes in their feelings about themselves and their bodies. The disease, which can alter physical appearance and abilities, bodily functions, and activities of living, can also damage a person's self-image. These changes can easily affect one's sex life. The person who no longer sees him- or herself as healthy, active, or intact may have difficulty having sexual feelings or feeling sexually attractive. In our culture sex is closely associated with health and vigor. Sexual activities may at first seem incompatible with illness even if there is little disability.

Some individuals report that at times they feel remote from their own bodies, as though the disabled limbs could not possibly be part of them. In these instances the person's body image is not fully integrated with his or her physical state; s/he may feel sexual or aroused but be unable to believe or accept that disability and sex can go together.

Social changes that can occur with MS (such as unemployment, divorce, or increased dependence) may be reflected in a lowering of self-esteem, which in turn may contribute to sexual difficulties. Any individuals, disabled or not, can experience sexual difficulties during periods when they do not feel good about themselves or their bodies. Self-esteem can also be affected by sexual performance; being able to perform satisfactorily in their sexual role plays an important part in determining how adult men and women feel about themselves. For many individuals, sexual gratification comes as much from "performing" well and pleasing a partner as it does from having an orgasm. People with MS and their partners frequently need to redefine what it means to "perform" well. Otherwise, they may become so worried about their ability to be adequate, attractive sexual partners that they shy away from intimate contact, convinced that they are no longer desirable.

In addition to changes in an individual's self-image and self-esteem, alterations frequently occur in interpersonal relationships. Two primary types of change are reported by families to cause a significant amount of stress: those related to gender roles, and those related to "caretaking" activities. For some families, traditional gender roles are highly valued and not easily changed. If the husband becomes unable to continue as breadwinner, or a wife cannot carry out her chosen activities inside and outside the home, these changes may be perceived as a loss of masculinity or femininity. The individuals may feel inadequate in their chosen roles, and this may carry over into their feelings about their sexual attractiveness. A spouse may also perceive the disabled partner as less masculine or feminine and therefore less attractive because of the alteration in roles.

A second type of role change involves the able-bodied spouse who becomes a nurse for the MS partner. It is very difficult for some individuals to respond sexually to a partner they have recently dressed, carried to the bathroom, catheterized, or cleaned.

Negative, angry feelings, a frequent accompaniment of the role changes described here, can also interfere with satisfying sexual activity. The able-bodied spouse may resent the changes brought about in the family by MS and be quite angry about the role changes forced on all of them. He or she may feel guilty about having these feelings toward the handicapped partner and be unable to express them. The MS partner can become very anxious and angry about his or her increased dependence and fearful of abandonment by the spouse on whom s/he has become dependent. Frequently individuals with MS report increasing resentment toward the spouse who nurses them, and they hesitate to express these feelings because of their fears of abandonment. These unspoken feelings in both partners can obviously impede the expression of positive loving feelings.

Couples who are experiencing sexual difficulties frequently report that they have also become less affectionate or demonstrative with each other. Most often, the satisfaction derived from close physical contact is lost because of anger or anxiety around sexual problems or other negative life changes brought about by the MS. Resentment over changes in their sexual life and anxiety about the ability to perform or feel sexual can lead partners to pull away from one another. "If I can't have sex, why bother" is the kind of feeling that can develop. As a result, frustration over sexual problems is compounded by loneliness and a feeling of isolation.

Dealing with Psychological Factors

The psychological factors that interfere with sexual interest and performance (such as overwhelming depression or anger, reduced self-esteem, and anxiety about ability to perform) are relieved most effectively through psychotherapy. The therapy can occur on an individual basis or with couples or groups. The general applicability of psychotherapy for individuals with MS is reviewed in Chapter 12. Briefly, therapy helps persons with MS and their families acknowledge, mourn, and accept the losses imposed on their lives. In this ongoing process, depression, frustration, and anxiety are relieved, and the individuals learn how to cope more effectively, productively, and enjoyably with the everyday problems and unpredictability of MS.

Group therapy can be very helpful both for individuals who are part of a couple and those who are not. It offers the opportunity for peer support and the sharing of experiences and feelings. The most common themes around sexuality to emerge in groups include:

1. Can I still be sexually attractive to someone if I'm handicapped?

2. Is my sexuality determined by others' responses to me or my feelings about myself: does being handicapped make me less masculine or feminine?

3. Can I still be a satisfactory sex partner even if I can't perform as I used to or do not have the same level of sexual interest?

4. How will I deal with my sexual feelings if I do not have a sex partner?

Group members are usually quite relieved to discover that others share their problems and concerns. There is no one answer to any of these questions, and each individual develops his or her own answers within the supportive group settings.

In *couples therapy* pertaining to sexual problems, the partners are helped to talk more openly about their sexual interests and feelings (both loving and angry). The changes imposed by MS make it more important than usual for couples to be able to talk freely about what they want, what does or does not feel good, and what is sexually stimulating. Each partner needs to feel comfortable expressing these feelings and requests without fear of being criticized or abruptly rejected by the other. In the same way, each partner needs to feel free to say no—in a gentle and noncritical way—to requests or suggestions which are unappealing.

The emotional impact of MS may introduce worry, anxiety, or depression into daily living and into sexual interactions. These feelings can lead to temporary or long-term difficulties for any individual or couple. Communication between partners, which is more imperative in times of difficulty, often becomes impossible. Feelings of loss, anger, resentment, frustration, and uncertainty can burden each partner, rendering them unable or unwilling to be open about such problems.

It is important to emphasize that these feelings are common in even the most loving couples. The goal of couples' treatment is to bring the feelings out into the open, reassure the couple of the normality of these feelings, and help them to come to terms with the changes imposed on their relationship. If sexual intercourse ceases to be an option, this is a significant loss which must be recognized and mourned. The couple who can share this loss openly will more likely continue sharing physical closeness and begin exploring and experimenting with alternative ways of expressing loving feelings and giving each other pleasure and comfort.

SOCIAL PRESSURE

The neurological, physical, and psychological problems that have been discussed here result from bodily changes or emotional reactions experienced by the person with MS. This section deals with the problems that result from the reactions and attitudes of others. Although these problems can affect anyone with MS, particular attention is paid to unmarried people who are not involved in a long-term relationship.

The current social attitudes toward health and sexuality may create special problems for the unmarried person with MS. Coping and communication may be particularly difficult; rather than having to learn how to work with one other person in coping with sexual problems, the single person may need to cope alone or with a series of people. A dating couple will probably not have the same commitment to each other, to the relationship, or to family as a married couple. Although sexual problems can certainly cause significant stress or unhappiness for a married couple, there may be greater motivation to overcome or overlook them for the sake of preserving the family relationships. The unmarried individual, on the other hand, may fear that a successful, intimate relationship can never begin or continue.

Three questions are commonly asked by single men and women with MS:

"How do I meet people if I can't participate in many of the social activities that other singles enjoy?"

"Who will want to get involved in a long-term relationship with me and this disease?"

"When should I tell the other person about my MS?"

The major significance of these questions is that they are asked at one time or another by almost all MS patients. The answers to these questions vary tremendously from one individual to another.

Physical disability may indeed interfere with a person's chances of making social contacts at a singles bar or sports event. People whose choice of recreation involves primarily sports or other strenuous physical activity are *not* as likely to be attracted to someone who cannot participate in these activities as are people whose interests are less physical. There are, however, other ways of meeting people. Taking classes, joining clubs or religious organizations, pursuing one's career, or doing volunteer work are all ways in which many people with MS have found satisfying relationships. The important thing seems to be to participate in group activities that are not physically taxing and in which it is possible to become an active, contributing member. This gives others the opportunity to get acquainted and comfortable with a person apart from his or her disability. Discussion and support groups for the handicapped, such as those sponsored by many MS Society chapters, not only provide an opportunity for meeting people but also enable men and women to share ideas on how to meet others.

There is no doubt that the problems and uncertainties of MS will cause some potential partners to shy away from a long-term relationship. This will not be true of everyone, however. The disabled person too often falls into the trap of saying "Why should I try to meet anyone—who would want me anyway?" In other words, the person anticipates a negative response from others rather than taking a chance and waiting to see what happens. He or she withdraws from people and activities in order to avoid disappointment. A certain amount of unhappiness and rejection is unavoidable—as is true for anyone—so the best course may be for the handicapped individual to let others get to know and like him/her and then make their own decision. This will occur most successfully in those kinds of group activities in which MS interferes least.

How and when to tell others about the MS seems to be a difficult issue for many people. On the one hand, MS plays a significant role in one's life and emotions. It is difficult to lay the groundwork for a satisfying, meaningful relationship while hiding such an important aspect of one's life. On the other hand, many people fear that talking about the MS will cause the other person to run away before the relationship can even begin. There is no one correct solution to this dilemma, and each person must eventually sort it out for him- or herself. Sharing one's feelings about this issue with others who are handicapped can be reassuring; it helps the person to feel less alone with the problem and provides a chance to learn from others' experiences. The most important rule of thumb is that no two people respond to another's disability in exactly the same way. One or two rejections does not mean that another will necessarily follow.

For the severely disabled person, finding sexual partners can indeed be a significant problem. The person may be sexually interested but feel unattractive to potential partners. The feeling that one is unattractive, although often unwarranted and unrealistic, may nevertheless be strong. A disabled person who is unsuccessful with one sexual partner may become convinced that no one will ever again find him/her attractive. The unfortunate reality is that our culture places great value on youth and health in relation to sexuality. Given that this is so, the very disabled individual may indeed not be as sexually attractive to others as a nondisabled person might be. He or she may then need to deal with this loss and find alternatives, either in the form of increased, individual sexual activities such as masturbation or other interesting and satisfying nonsexual activities. Companionship and the sharing of common interests need not be lost simply because one is not involved in a sexual relationship. People who have a variety of interests and enjoy sharing them will always be valued by others. The challenge lies in finding practical and enjoyable ways of pursuing these activities, hobbies, or talents.

An additional word should be said about the possible problems confronted by gay men and women who have MS. They have great difficulty in finding help with sexual questions, either in the literature on disability, which tends to ignore the problems and needs of gay people, or from health professionals who may shy away from any issues related to homosexuality. Being a "minority within a minority" can make it doubly difficult to find the help and support one needs in dealing with sexual or any other kinds of problems.

Gay men and women will need to confront these difficulties head on if they are to find the support they need. Therapists, sex counselors, and health professionals who are comfortable with, and knowledgeable about, sexual difficulties, disability, and homosexuality can be found. Again, finding one unhelpful or rejecting professional does not mean that all will be that way.

CHILDBEARING AND BIRTH CONTROL

Fertility remains for the most part unimpaired in individuals with MS. Couples engaging in intercourse must make the same decisions about birth control as do individuals without neurological impairment. Any form of birth control which is effective and manageable is permitted with MS. Some women with weakness or tremor in the hands find the diaphragm to be cumbersome. Similarly, men with dexterity problems find it difficult to put on a condom. Such problems can be solved by having the partner insert the diaphragm or put on the condom as part of the sexual foreplay. Where such a solution is not practical or desirable, birth control pills or the IUD are usually acceptable means of birth control. Women who are experiencinig diminished sensation in the vaginal area should avoid using an IUD since they might be insensitive to slippage of the device.

The decision of whether to have children is a very personal one. There is *no medical reason* why an adult with MS should not become a parent. There is no evidence that MS causes any problems for the unborn or newborn child. The disease cannot be transmitted to the baby. In addition, there is very little evidence that the stress of childbirth has any lasting effects on the disease. Each couple must evaluate for themselves their feelings about childrearing and their ability to raise a child should the disability become severe.

SUMMARY

It is clear that sexual problems related to MS can take many forms and affect many areas of the sexual relationship. These problems are compounded by the difficulties individuals and couples have in discussing their concerns with each other and their doctors. This chapter will hopefully serve to reassure a person with MS that he or she is not alone with these problems. The knowledgeable health care professional or family or sex therapist is available to provide help and support with this adjustment. Likewise, spouse, lover, or friends may be crucial. Sexual feelings and their enjoyment can continue to be an important part of living and relating even if the mode of sexual expression requires some adjustment.

12

Psychological Changes

Nicholas LaRocca, Rosalind Kalb, and Seymour R. Kaplan

Scientists have searched in vain for an "MS personality." If such a personality existed, it would either predispose a person to develop MS or else it would bear the "stamp" of the disease after symptoms developed. Hysteria, for example, was advanced as a personality pattern that might in part cause MS. The two disorders were often linked in the past because of the difficulty in distinguishing between them. Early signs of MS (such as loss of sensation, weakness, and visual changes) resemble many of the symptoms of hysteria. Emotional factors in the hysteric were thought to cause changes in the blood vessels of the nervous system. These blood vessel changes, in turn, were regarded as one of the causes of demyelination (the nerve sheath changes that cause MS).

Today, hysteria is no longer regarded as typical of people who have MS, and modern diagnostic procedures make confusion between them less likely. In fact, most authorities believe that there is no such thing as an "MS-prone personality."

DO EMOTIONS CAUSE MS?

The demise of the notion of the MS personality has by no means ended speculation on the contribution of the emotions to causing MS. Psychologial stress (loss of a loved one, migration, etc.) has long been suggested as a cause of MS. Most people with MS find that emotional pressures do cause a temporary worsening in their symptoms. However, does stress actually accelerate the development of the disease or hasten its course? These longstanding questions received international attention when Richard Queen, a U.S.

State Department employee, developed MS during his stressful captivity by Iranians in Teheran.

If stress does play a role in MS it is probably a minor role, operating in conjunction with biological factors such as a slow virus and/or an autoimmune response (Chapter 2). In other words, when the physical conditions for the development of the disease already exist, stress may increase the likelihood that the individual will develop the disease. In people who already have MS, stress may slightly increase the frequency and severity of exacerbations (flare-ups of the disease). Scientific evidence for such effects are very sketchy at present. More research is needed to determine if stress plays a role in MS. In the meantime, stress should be regarded as a normal feature of living. Many useful strategies exist for coping with stress (such as hypnosis, relaxation, meditation, and biofeed-back). Although there is no proof that stress management techniques have any effect on MS, they do contribute to a sense of well-being and are generally harmless. Certainly no one with MS should attempt to manage stress by avoiding stressful situations altogether—that could mean renouncing life almost completely.

DOES MS CAUSE EMOTIONAL CHANGES?

Damage done to the brain by MS can result in personality changes. It is not clear, however, if there is any consistent pattern of changes caused by MS. One change that is occasionally seen in MS is known as "emotional incontinence." In such instances a person may laugh or cry very easily and with little or no provocation. Shifts from happiness to sadness are rapid and unpredictable. Such behavior is rare in MS and is sometimes misinterpreted as schizophrenia, to which it is unrelated. Over the years, most speculation has centered on two other personality changes. The first is lability (a volatility or instability in the emotions), and the second is euphoria (an abnormal sense of well-being). At one time these changes were regarded as typical of MS. Plaque formation (lesions) that damages areas of the brain that normally inhibit emotions were thought to be responsible. Lability and euphoria both seem to be more frequent among those people with MS who are the most disabled and who also have some loss of mental acuity. The evidence, however, is not conclusive.

Modern studies have generally found that depression, not euphoria or lability, is the most striking feature of the person with MS. Often people who make apparently "euphoric" statements report that they really feel depressed. Their "false optimism" seems to function as an important part of their coping strategy. Euphoria and lability do exist in MS but are probably less important and less frequent than once supposed. It is also not clear if they are an emotional reaction to the physical effects of MS, or if they are a result of damage to the nervous system.

To summarize, it appears that there is no such thing as a "typical MS personality." Instead, the personality of the person with MS is determined by pre-MS influences (such as genetics, family relationships, and culture). Similarities do exist, however, in the ways that people react to the disease, as MS often presents different people with a similar set of challenges.

SHARED EXPERIENCES

MS is a unique disease carrying with it a special set of conditions which help to shape how individuals feel emotionally. To the extent that different people share this same set of conditions, their reactions may have a great deal in common. This is not to say that there is an MS personality, rather that people with MS often have many shared experiences. MS is usually disabling in terms of a person's ability to function; this is due to changes in strength, endurance, vision, mobility, coordination, and sexual response. The vast majority of people who get MS have their first symptoms between the ages of 20 and 50. During this period of life, people have often attained some career goals and are in the midst of family, social, and job responsibilities. Painful adjustment to changes in family life and work, reduced independence, and a curtailed level of participation may be necessary. Changes in family roles may occur as loved ones adjust to the physical and emotional realities of a chronic, progressive, and disabling illness.

The effects of the disease are frequently unstable. Disability is likely to progress, and changes are unpredictable. It is almost impossible to foretell the occurrence, severity, or consequences of attacks. Not knowing how the disease will behave can be a great source of anxiety. The changing nature of MS requires continual readjustment throughout life. The next part of this chapter is devoted to the crucial question of how people manage to adjust to the pervasive and unpredictable effects of MS, and what sources of help are available.

ADJUSTING TO MS

The major psychological question of MS is: "How do people adjust to MS?" Adjustment consists of all the ways in which a person responds to the illness in thought, feeling, and action. If MS were an invisible condition producing neither disability nor threat of future harm, there would be no need for adjustment. Because MS has widespread effects, it requires a great deal of adjustment.

The most important effects of MS occur in three areas. First and foremost are the well-known effects of demyelination (a form of nerve damage) on such basic physical functions as walking, sight, speech, eye–hand coordination, sexual performance, and bladder control. Next come the extensive psychological effects the disease may have on the person with MS. These include threats to self-esteem, uncertainty about the future, and feelings of helplessness. Finally, MS can have many social effects. Examples would be loss of job, changes in friendships, and shifts in family roles. All of these effects demand some response, and most have in common the need to adapt to change—sometimes dramatic change.

When looking at adjustment, two important questions arise. The first concerns the events that unfold as the person with MS adjusts. What tasks must be accomplished in the process of adjustment? The second question concerns the conditions helping or hindering adjustment. Why do some people adjust better than others?

Adjustment is such an individualized process that there is some danger in trying to summarize it. In MS particularly, no two people have the same symptoms. Personalities, jobs, and families differ enormously. As a result, no two people adjust at the same speed or in exactly the same way. However, work with people who have MS has shown that many do share similar experiences. Although each person is unique, everyone should find a bit of their own experiences reflected in what follows.

THE PROCESS OF ADJUSTMENT

In recent years it has become popular to look at adjustment (to any situation) as a series of stages or major tasks that unfold in some regular order. This approach has been applied to MS and provides a convenient way to trace a person's progress from the appearance of symptoms through the entire process of adjustment. Naturally, people differ in their progress through these stages. Some progress faster than others. Many linger for a time at one stage or another. Some may skip stages or combine two stages into one. Still others tackle the stages in a different order. Nevertheless, for most individuals, adjusting to MS is characterized by the following four stages: uncertainty, acceptance, adaptation, and emergence.

Uncertainty

After symptoms of MS first appear and before a diagnosis is made, uncertainty may predominate. During this period the person with MS may feel nervous and confused. The major task that seems to face people during this period is to resolve the questions: "What is wrong with me, and what is going to happen?" On the average it takes around 3 years to establish a diagnosis of MS. As a result, this stage can be a long and difficult one. A brief history illustrates the stages the affected person must go through:

A 35-year-old married mother of two who works as a guidance counselor has enjoyed robust health all her life, with rarely a day sick. She wakes up one morning with an almost imperceptible numbness and weakening of her legs. Attributing it to overwork, she ignores it. When it gets worse, she goes to her family doctor who refers her to a neurologist. At this point she begins to wonder if she has a brain tumor. A friend tells her that "It's all in your mind."

The neurologist orders several tests including a myelogram, a CAT scan, spinal tap, and blood tests. Some of these tests are not very pleasant. All the tests come out normal, and gradually the numbness and weakness disappear. The neurologist cannot give her a diagnosis and advises her to call if her symptoms return.

Life returns almost to normal except for a nagging uncertainty: "What's wrong with me? Will all this happen again?" A year later the numbness and weakness appear again, but this time accompanied by blurred vision in both eyes. Another trip to the neurologist is followed by more tests including a new one, the visual evoked potential test (Chapter 3). This time the doctor is certain—it is MS. Finally, knowing what is wrong brings a sense of relief. MS is not a very familiar disease but at least it does not sound fatal.

This young woman's struggle with uncertainty did not last as long as that of some. Approximately half of the people who get MS are not diagnosed until 2 years after their first trip to a doctor. If this woman's diagnosis had not been established after her second attack, she could have gone on wondering about the cause of her problems. Advances in diagnostic procedures make it easier to identify MS than ever before. Nevertheless, diagnostic euphemisms such as "autoimmune disease" and "virus of the nervous system" are still in use. Reluctance on the part of doctor or family to disclose the diagnosis can needlessly prolong and intensify uncertainty. Lack of appropriate information can also hurt. Uncertainty may arise from not knowing the important features of the disease: what it does and does not do. It is probably easier for most people to adjust to something if they know what it is they are adjusting to. Knowing about the symptoms, course, complications, and treatment are all important items to know.

During this and all subsequent stages, finding good medical care is essential. Sources of information are also crucial. Health care professionals may be the main source of such information. Books, articles, conferences, and the local chapter of the MS Society are also valuable sources of knowledge. Knowing more about the disease can help to dispel destructive misconceptions while allowing the person to assume an active and effective role in his or her own medical care and prevention of complications.

When symptoms first appear, many people encounter problems with family or friends who believe that: "It's all in your mind." Loved ones may hope that by maintaining normal activities the strange problems and symptoms will go away. This attitude may be especially common before the diagnosis is established. It is easier to think that someone you love has a passing emotional problem than a chronic physical disease. In the early stages of the disease, a supportive rather than skeptical attitude on the part of loved ones would be helpful but is not always easy to achieve.

In MS uncertainty is not just an initial stage of the illness. In a sense, the uncertainty never ends. The changeable and unpredictable nature of the illness guarantees a degree of uncertainty throughout life. Future plans may be cast into doubt. Should work continue as before or be curtailed? Should the family move to a more accessible house or stay put? Conflicting advice will be in ample supply while certainty remains elusive.

Acceptance

Once the diagnosis of MS has been established, acceptance of the disease and of its effects becomes a major issue. During this time, the person with MS may experience a wide range of feelings including shock, disbelief, denial, confusion, nervousness, and anger. The major task facing people at this stage is the intellectual and emotional acceptance of the reality of chronic illness.

There is little in the experience of most people to prepare them to cope with a chronic illness. Most people are accustomed to good health and come to expect it. Most of us develop a feeling of invulnerability: "It won't happen to me!" After the diagnosis is made, questions such as "Is this really happening to me?" of "Why me?" are asked by many people. The former feeling of security has been stripped away, leaving a sense of vulnerability, like one who has suddenly been victimized. It is similar to the feeling people get when they first discover their house has been burglarized. After-ward, danger seems uncomfortably close.

At this point it is possible to forget that you have MS. It is like a bad dream. It is fair to say that most people experience some difficulty in accepting the disease and denial is to be expected. Having a chronic illness is a painful reality that often needs to be held at a safe distance by means of denial. Doing so can aid ad-justment by helping the person cope with upsetting feelings. Denial can take many forms—some helpful, some not so helpful. Some people engage in a harried search for the cure that always seems just over the horizon. Others find it difficult to be around other people with MS or to even discuss the disease.

People sometimes linger at this stage. Some practically stop living while they wait for the elusive cure. They may reject vocational rehabilitation, counseling, physical therapy, and even the use of a cane. Their one hope is to be restored to health and full functioning. As a result, they are unable to acknowledge the reality of having MS.

Acceptance is difficult in part because it implies coming to grips with change. Everyday habits and abilities may have to be altered. Although change can be exciting, forced change due to loss is painful and upsetting. Moreover, most people benefit from a degree of stability and familiarity in their lives. When the boat begins to rock, we hang on all the more strongly.

The anger and frustration attending acceptance may be directed against the doctor. He or she may be seen as meddlesome at one time and indifferent at another. Likewise, family members may be looked upon as either overprotective or uncaring. Loved ones may feel as if nothing they say comes out quite right, and the level of tension around the person with MS rises. It is important to remember that many of these emotional ups and downs are quite common and constitute a very normal part of the adjustment process.

Professionals, family, and friends can assist by helping to create an atmosphere conducive to growth. Communicating a reasonable optimism is essential. Having MS is no picnic, but it is not the end of the world either. Appropriate information should be available when the person with MS is ready to use it. However, not everyone wants a flood of facts right away. Many people need time to get used to the idea of having MS before they feel comfortable learning about the disease. They should not be rushed. A supportive, trusting environment where there is room for the MS person's feelings can help growth and change to proceed more smoothly.

Adaptation

Once acceptance has begun and some degree of change has taken place, adaptation begins. During this period the person's reactions vary widely and may include shifts in self-concept and body image, nervousness, anger, and depression. The task facing people in this stage is the preservation of the quality of life while incorporating into everyday living the physical, psychological, and social changes due to MS.

What are these changes and what do they mean to the person?

Physical change is the most direct and obvious result of MS. Physical abilities may be reduced. For example, loss of some or all ability to walk curtails mobility and independence. New ways of doing things must be learned. Restricted activities may ensue. Other physical changes may include loss of stamina, tremors, painful muscle spasms, loss of bladder control, and disruption of the sexual response. All add up to a potential reduction in the range and frequency of activities once taken for granted. These facts, however, do not add up to the end of living.

Psychological effects seem to follow upon the physical changes. Loss of abilities and physical restrictions put strain on the way a person is able to view him- or herself. Pride in and satisfaction with self may be reduced. Moreover, the person with MS may be isolated from many of the people and events that serve to bolster self-esteem. Feelings of helplessness and impotence can further erode a once strong sense of self. Society's emphasis on independence and self-reliance can even encourage guilt feelings in someone forced by MS to rely on others.

Some changes in values may take place. Old ways of evaluating one's worth (physical strength, stamina) may give way to new ones (communication skills, intellectual ability). Although unexpected resources may be discovered, the process can be a painful one. Plans and expectations may go up in smoke as life takes a new and unexpected turn. Self-concept is shaken but eventually steadies. The person with MS is able to feel good about him- or herself while accepting the limitations imposed by the disease.

Many feelings sweep across a person's life at this stage. Guilt may appear as the person sees him- or herself as a burden on others. Physical imperfection may be subconsciously regarded as a sign of moral imperfection. Society may encourage such feelings by its tendency to stigmatize the disabled. Feelings of loss and depression may be quite strong. The individual goes through a long and painful process of grieving for lost abilities and experiences.

In addition to physical and psychological changes, significant social changes are often a part of MS. Families are usually unprepared to deal with chronic illness. Loss of abilities and reduced independence may lead to a shift in roles—in who is expected to do what in the family. Anger and sadness concerning these changes can hinder communication in the family if they go unexpressed. Family members may have trouble knowing if they are doing too little or too much for the person with MS, and the person with MS may be unsure of how much help he or she wants or needs. Family plans and everyday habits may have to change. Sexual difficulties brought on by MS may lead to a reduction in the frequency and satisfaction of sexual relations. The person with MS may become more dependent on the able-bodied family members. This increased dependency may develop into a partial merging of identities. The person with MS thinks of the able-bodied person as an extension of himself rather than as a completely separate person.

Friendships are also affected by MS. Marginal friends may lose interest if the person with MS is no longer able to travel as easily to parties and other social events. The reduction in shared experiences can open a gap between friends. Some acquaintances may focus on the disability and lose sight of the person. Others may feel awkward, not knowing "how to act." Spontaneity can suffer. Of course, close friends are likely to overcome these obstacles, and such relationships may grow.

For single persons, MS may bring special problems. Opportunities to meet new people may be curtailed. When opportunities do arise, the effects of the disease on spontaneity and attitudes of the able-bodied may interfere with the development of new relationships.

Work and education can also be seriously affected by MS. Architectural barriers and transportation problems can make school and working impractical at best. Accomodations in the workplace or school (such as ramps) or transfer to a job with different physical demands can help to minimize disruption in these important areas of living. Particularly crucial is the need for co-workers, employers, teachers, and fellow students to have an informed and understanding attitude toward the disabled.

Throughout adaptation, the person with MS is assessing the many changes brought on by the illness in terms of their personal and practical meaning. During this period people with MS tackle the most critical emotional task involved in adjustment—grieving. Grieving for lost abilities and experiences begins as soon as MS produces its first limitations. However, grief cannot occur until some acceptance of the reality of the disease takes place. For example, some people never fully grieve the death of a loved one. They were never able to grieve because they never really accepted the death. In MS, grief reaches an intense point after acceptance begins. The process of grieving may subside after a time but probably never ends completely.

Grief is one of the most painful of human emotions to feel or to witness in others. The sadness, anger, and despair involved in grief are difficult for most of us to deal with. However, of all the painful human experiences, grief is one of the most healing. For those who can successfully grieve a loss, the result is emergence with a sense of relief, peace, and resolution.

Mourning for losses in MS takes place alongside the struggle to learn and to adapt. Alterations take place in how the person sees him- or herself. New ideas, new feelings, new techniques are tried. Some are discarded, and others are incorporated into everyday life.

The person strives to accept realistically the limitations of the illness while making the most of remaining abilities. Eventually, MS and its many changes are successfully woven into the fabric of everyday life.

Emergence

Once necessary accomodations in life style have been made, emergence can take place. During this period, the person with MS may experience a lessening of nervousness and anger as a widening of perspective takes place. In many people mild or intermittent depression may continue as grieving for lost abilities and activities proceeds. The major task that seems to be accomplished during this period is placing of the illness in perspective as the person with MS carries on with everyday life.

Physical, emotional, and social changes have been met and in-tegrated as well as possible into the individual's life style. MS now begins to occupy less time, less attention, and less energy. The regular business of living more and more commands its proper attention. As life goes on, MS is never completely forgotten, but it does shrink in importance as other features of life grow in sig-nificance.

Adaptation is not a process that occurs once and then is over forever. The process is an ongoing one. Keeping life changes and the sense of self intact requires constant investments of energy. Adjustment is a lifelong process.

The initial period is probably the toughest and requires the most from the person. Once that painstaking initial work has been done, there seems to be more of the person available to meet the usual joys and sorrows, pleasures, and challenges of life. At this point, the person with MS has constructed a new life and is ready to carry on with the business of living. He or she feels more in control of things and better able to exercise options in social and family life. As emergence proceeds, depression may remain. Sadness may wax and wane as symptoms change and with the ordinary frustrations of living.

Emergence is often a time for making contingency plans. Future problems can be anticipated, particularly if the disease is stable. For instance, people may make "what if" plans. Thoughts may run through the mind such as: "What will I do if I can no longer get around with a walker? Maybe I could look into the costs of ramping the backdoor, just in case." Modifications in the house and work that were begun earlier may be extended or further modifications considered. Such planning is not an expression of pessimism. Rather, preparing mentally for realistic possibilities enables the person to feel less helpless when and if things do change adversely. Having some plans worked out ahead of time gives one a psychological edge. Nothing is more devastating than an unpleasant surprise. Danger is less frightening if one is prepared for it. Preparation involves knowing what might happen and planning what to do about it.

At times the future may seem overwhelming and foreboding. Then a useful strategy may be to take each day as an individual challenge to be met, regardless of what happens or does not happen in the future. This strategy divides the seemingly immense task of living into more manageable units. Sudden changes, though, may find the person totally unprepared and take a greater than necessary toll.

Family and friends are crucial to emergence. They can support the MS person's struggle to "normalize" living without catering to unrealistic expectations. A good working relationship with a medical team can also help. By keeping physical problems under control, more attention can be devoted to living. In all relationships, a comfortable balance might be struck between accepting help and doing things independently. As emergence takes place, the self, the world, and the disease are all in proper perspective and life can go on.

And Yet Again

When symptoms get worse or disability increases, new demands for adjustment occur. At such times the prior stages of adjustment may be relived. Many of the same reactions take place, ranging from disbelief through anger, nervousness, depression, and changes in self-concept.

After the first emergence and when the disease is stable, things may be pretty much under control for the person with MS. Work, social life, and family life are changed but proceeding on a new and satisfactory level. Then an exacerbation occurs. At first there may be uncertainty. "Is this really an attack or am I just tired?" Acceptance again becomes an issue as the person is faced with a new level of limitation. Acceptance can take some time as hope lingers that a remission will take place. New adaptations may be necessary, such as moving from a cane to a walker or from full to part-time employment. Eventually these new accommodations can be made, and the individual emerges again to carry on the business of living.

Does adjustment go easier the second time? Each person is different in regard to ease of adjusting. The second attack can be very devastating emotionally. After the initial attack, one naturally hopes that there will be no more. The second attack dashes such hopes for many people. After their second attack it beomes harder to believe that another will not take place.

Continuing adjustment is complicated by the peculiarities of MS. Other illnesses may mimic an attack. A bout with the flu may come and go. When a real attack of MS occurs, it is difficult to believe that it will not go away as the flu did. The unpredictability and changeability of MS can confuse. After one attack complete remission may occur, whereas after another little or no improvement may follow.

Of course, improvements can and do occur. A lessening or disappearance of symptoms may reverse previous changes in life style. Self-esteem may recover some of its old supports. If the disease is very stable, a stable adjustment may result. For most people, though, MS is a progressive condition. As symptoms progress, so can adjustment. Even when disability is severe, a satisfying life is possible.

HELPING AND HINDERING ADJUSTMENT

Having seen how adjustment proceeds, the question remains: What are the conditions that help or hinder adjustment? People differ tremendously in how rapidly they adjust to the disease, how easily the process goes, and how comfortable that adjustment eventually is. When explaining why these differences exist, three influences seem to be important: the individual, the environment, and the disease itself.

The Individual

The most important influence on adjustment is probably what the person possesses as an individual to deal with the problems brought on by MS. These resources of the individual might be called "coping ability." Richard Lazarus of the University of California has described coping as possessing two main functions: reducing tension and solving problems. Reducing tension involves keeping emotions within limits a person can live with and tolerate. Problem solving involves actually searching for workable solutions to difficulties brought about by the illness.

Different coping strategies may be used in different situations. Sometimes problem solving cannot proceed until tension is reduced. Three familiar coping strategies are: denial, giving up, and problem solving.

In denial, a problem is dealt with by not acknowledging its presence. The person with unrealistic expectations who tries to do too much, who avoids other people with MS, or who cannot talk about MS is probably using an exaggerated form of denial. Denial is helpful in reducing tension or dealing with an impossible situation, but it rarely solves problems. At times denial is necessary for everyone, and adjustment might be more difficult without it. We all use denial at one time or another. Sometimes denial is conscious. Thinking about an upcoming examination makes you nervous, and so you try not to think about it. Denial can also operate subconsciously with the person not even aware that he or she is blocking something out. If problems are to be tackled on a long-term basis, coping probably has to progress beyond denial.

Giving up contrasts with denial and is similar to adopting the "sick role." Someone who has given up leads a life unnecessarily centered around MS. Abilities are not fully utilized. Excessive dependency, frequent calls to the doctor, and withdrawal from normal activities that can still be performed are all signs of giving up. Like denial, giving up may have its time and place. Also like denial, it does little to solve the problems created by MS. Although there may be times when giving up is the most workable alternative, it usually carries with it unnecessary disability.

Active problem solving consists of neither denying the illness nor giving up. Rather, bad feelings and physical limits are acknowledged while remaining abilities are utilized. Help and support are accepted without overdependency. The problems presented by the disease are confronted and a try is made at solving them.

People with a positive image of themselves, who feel good about themselves, seem to be less threatened by problems and better able to solve them. Such people are confident of their ability to tackle a challenge. The realistic and independent person who accepts rather than avoids challenge may therefore fare better emotionally. Past handling of crises and problems is a good indication of how well coping will proceed, as these abilities have been developed slowly and over a lifetime. Effective communication skills (getting one's message across and having it accepted by others) can help the individual make full use of outside support and resources. Intelligence, education, and financial security can all make a big difference in how well the person deals with the disease, though they can never make up for a lack of coping skills. Finally, the way the person sees the disease can make a big difference. Adjusting to MS as a physical disability is probably easier than adjusting to MS as a sign of moral weakness. In this regard, how one sees the disease is affected to a great extent by influences within the environment.

The Environment

Family and friends can alter the impact of MS by direct help and indirectly by modifying the way the person views the disease. Common forms of direct help are financial support and sharing tasks. Indirect forms of assistance include helping the person with MS to utilize their own assets in coping. One such asset, self-esteem, can be enhanced tremendously through social support. Self-esteem is aided by relating to the person as a responsible, capable adult regardless of the disability. Attitudes of family and friends toward the illness will influence the person with MS. If other people see MS as a challenge rather than as a devastation or as emotional weakness, it may help the person with MS in maintaining a realistic and workable view of the disease. The tendency of the person with MS to use denial, giving up, or problem solving will be affected by the coping style that significant others use and encourage.

Family and friends can be most helpful under certain conditions. Social support that is geographically near is more useful than support that is very real but distant. Significant others with many ties to the community may be more helpful because they are in a position to tap sources of help outside the person's immediate circle. It is most helpful if MS is not allowed to become the centerpiece of family life or of friendships. Each family member should be able to retain a degree of independence and the opportunity to lead their own lives. Flexibility and the ability to deal with change are crucial along with a varied supply of coping strategies. Most important is a supportive atmosphere in which communication is open, clear, and free of conflicting messages. Ability to air problems and feelings and to try out new ideas in a noncritical environment are essential to adjustment.

Professional help also has an important place. Medical care can establish an active stance toward the disease which carries over into everyday life. It also serves to avoid unnecessary disability by preventing and promptly treating complications. Knowledge gained from professionals helps to dispel feelings of impotence and uncertainty. Reassurance, support, and understanding can all be provided by professionals. Perhaps most importantly, professionals influence attitudes toward the disease and the self. Realistic optimism combined with an active, problem-solving attitude can boost adjustment. Also essential is an attitude of respect for the person as a responsible, capable adult.

One area of professional service is especially useful. Psychotherapy or counseling, particularly in groups, can have many benefits. It helps to mobilize diffuse anger, often turning it into useful assertiveness. The "sick role" can be challenged by other group members who have MS and who therefore speak with more authority than someone without a disability. Group members share fears and explore behaviors that are stumbling blocks to adjustment. The group can provide an atmosphere of trust, acceptance, and understanding in which new behavior patterns can be tried out. Skills in social encounters may become less awkward. Positive qualities of the individual are bolstered by the closeness and mutual regard of the group and by the respect of the therapist. Rap groups, less formal than psychotherapy and often with a changing membership, can also be useful in airing feelings and exchanging information. Such groups, however, do not delve deeply into the issues involved in living with a chronic illness.

The wider community is also significant in adjustment. Religion, for instance, can provide social support while helping people to find philosophical meaning in their lives. Local attitudes toward the disabled can help life move more smoothly if such attitudes are informed and supportive. Employers who give fair treatment to handicapped workers can make a big difference. Appropriate accommodations in the work place are often crucial. Individuals in white-collar occupations, who have greater flexibility in time and control over their own work, have a definite edge. Community groups can be of great assistance. Among the most important of these is the National Multiple Sclerosis Society. The MS Society and its local chapters offer a number of services important to the person with MS. Research that may eventually lead to a treatment or prevention for MS is supported by the Society. Local chapters often sponsor clinics or else can refer people to medical facilities. Recreational programs are often a part of the chapter's services. Rap groups are offered by many chapters. Information is available on subjects ranging from research to transportation. The Society provides an invaluable opportunity to meet and talk to other people who also live with MS and understand its challenges.

Many community agencies provide practical help to the person with MS. Vocational rehabilitation agencies can assist with education, job training, or placement. Service groups such as the Multiple Sclerosis Service Organization can assist with physical and recreational needs. The visiting nurse service may provide certain types of medical care in the home under a physician's supervision. Government offices for the handicapped often sponsor meetings on issues concerning the disabled. They sometimes fund transportation or training programs. Speaking to other disabled people will help to determine the availability of many of these often obscure but valuable agencies.

The Disease

Adjusting to MS is adjusting to an illness with many faces. Some of these faces are easier to deal with than others. MS usually appears between the ages of 20 and 50. For those who get it very early in life, education and career plans may be seriously disrupted. Those who get it very late in life may have grown children and are at a point where they can retire early without significant loss of income. People who have the disease for a longer period of time are frequently better adjusted than those who have it only a short time. It takes time to learn how to deal with MS and so the person newly diagnosed may not be coping as well as they will a few years later.

Different symptoms present widely different challenges. The inability to walk is visible and understandable to others. Weakness and fatigue, on the other hand, are often misinterpreted as laziness or depression. Urinary symptoms may make one very self-concious socially even if they are not very disabling physically. Sexual problems may be invisible to others but very disruptive for the person's love life.

The features of MS most decisive for adjustment are probably the severity and course of the disease. It is more difficult to adjust to a severe impairment because of the greater change involved. Yet the person with very mild disability is at a special disadvantage.

The mildly disabled person may look "well" and may be perceived by others as having nothing wrong. Nevertheless, such a person may be unable to do everything he or she once did. People seem capable of adjusting well to all levels of disability, even the very severe, especially if the disease remains stable. It is the unpredictable and changeable nature of the illness which really challenges adjustment. Living with uncertainty and repeated change represents an enormous strain on one's coping ability.

SUMMARY

Emotions do not appear to cause MS. Emotional stress may contribute in a small way to MS, but there does not seem to be a "typical" personality more likely to get MS. The disease may produce some personality changes due to neurological damage, but these seem insignificant when compared to the effects of MS on walking, vision, etc. MS also does not seem to produce an "MS personality." However, people with MS do have a lot in common. They are all faced with the need to adjust to changeable, unpredictable, chronic, disabling disease.

Adjustment begins with the need to resolve the uncertainty produced by the first appearance of symptoms. Once a diagnosis is made, acceptance of the reality of having MS and all it implies can take place. Adaptation follows as the person with MS grieves for what has been lost and builds a new and different way of life. Once adaptation has occurred, MS may fade into the background a bit as the person with MS carries on the business of living.

The process of adjustment is affected by an individual's own coping ability, by aspects of their environment, and by characteristics of the disease. No two people adjust in the same way or at the same pace. Nevertheless, adjustment can be very successful, and the quality of life can remain quite good in spite of the tremendous challenges presented by MS.

13

Social Adaptations

Nancy J. Holland, Lola Sprinzeles, and Seymour R. Kaplan

The diagnosis of a chronic disease necessitates varying degrees of adaptive changes in all areas of living. Social adaptation to MS involves the assessment and possible readjustment of life style, role expectations, and goals. This process can be difficult and confusing as the uncertainty of MS creates potential obstacles to every decision. Despite these difficulties, people living with MS need to examine important relationships, explore their options, and identify those situations where personal control can be exerted. The intent of this chapter is to increase awareness of areas to be explored and to encourage constructive planning.

A few points should be noted before proceeding. Psychological factors and responses (such as depression) overlap in many ways with social or relationship issues. These are discussed in Chapter 12. Likewise, sexuality is an important component of intimate relationships, and discussion of this area is concentrated in Chapter 11. Finally, many broad guidelines are stated here. It is well to remember that they are generalizations and so are not "right" for everyone. Thus they are best approached as ideas for consideration, not as directives. The individual with MS, or a family member, must be the ultimate determinant of his or her attitudes and actions.

INTERPERSONAL RELATIONSHIPS

Individuals with MS generally experience anxiety about interpersonal relationships at some point following diagnosis. To tell or not to tell, how and when to tell, what information to communicate—these questions pertain not only to the newly diagnosed but to the majority of people with MS who have minimal visible dysfunction.

195

Family members have similar concerns but may have emotional responses which are different from those of the person with MS such as guilt about good health or anger at life changes imposed by the chronic disease. These and other commonly encountered inter-personal difficulties are addressed in this section.

THE NEWLY DIAGNOSED PATIENT

Following diagnosis, much psychic energy is concentrated on integrating this new and frightening entity into one's concept of self. The impulse may be to inform everyone—an attempt to control reality by controlling the information communicated. Conversely, some people try to make MS "go away" by not discussing it with anyone. Neither extreme is helpful, and middle-ground responses can be achieved. In addition, both the MS individual and family feel frightened, sad, angry, or optimistic, but not necessarily in concert with each other. Dealing with this range of emotions, while continuing with normal activities of daily living, can only be de-scribed as very difficult and stressful. Although each situation is different and must be evaluated independently, some guidelines formulated from ongoing counseling with MS clients may be useful.

1. *Sharing information and feelings about a new MS diagnosis with "significant others"* (spouse, parents, roommate) generally releases pent-up emotions, relieves some feelings of aloneness, and allows those closest to be involved. Strong feelings are rarely ef-fectively concealed, and the attempt to do so may alienate those with whom a loving and trusting relationship already exists.

2. *General disclosure to peripheral people* tends to increase anx-iety at this point because repeated explanations are needed, and the fear of rejection usually accompanies each announcement. Also the response of casual acquaintances may be more curiosity than con-cern. The emotional turbulence present following diagnosis makes such indiscriminate disclosure especially problematic.

3. *Grieving* is expected following diagnosis of a chronic illness such as MS. Spouses or others with a close emotional relationship may undergo a similar response. Communication during this time helps both parties and can actually strengthen the relationship.

4. *For those involved in dating situations*, disclosure of MS best occurs after a comfortable rapport has been established. This may be the first meeting or the tenth—whenever the relationship progresses toward emotional intimacy. Fear of the partner's response does not disappear or even diminish with time, as potential rejection is painful under any circumstances. Therefore waiting for a totally comfortable moment will undoubtedly prolong anxiety within the relationship.

5. *Plans for the future* can be made optimistically, as most people with MS do not become severely disabled. However, "plan for the worst—hope for the best" is a good maxim to follow. For example, consider potential disability when a move to a new home is being planned. Hopefully, the need for structural accessibility will never materialize; but should disability occur, environmental barriers in the home will be one less problem with which to contend.

6. *Pregnancy* is not believed to affect the course of MS, and MS is not hereditary. Family planning can be guided by pre-existing criteria, with some attention to the possible future disability of the MS parent.

7. *Gaining greater understanding of MS* by reading relevant material and questioning experienced health professionals usually increases the sense of control over the disease. Reducing the unknown to a known entity usually reduces the fear.

8. *When one becomes aware of the MS, most individuals and families experience varied and intense emotional responses.* They may perceive some of these feelings as being "bad" or "negative," depending on their upbringing and value systems. It is important for all concerned to understand that feelings themselves are neither good nor bad in the moral sense, although some are undeniably pleasant, whereas others are extremely painful. Moral judgment implies choice, whereas feelings simply emerge unsolicited by the individual. If feelings could be chosen, it is likely that joy and contentment would be prime selections. This concept is crucial when dealing with the emotional upheaval following an MS diagnosis, as feelings such as anger and depression are normal, appropriate, and understandable. Difficulties arise when feelings such as these are

denied or misdirected, particularly because the obvious target is loved ones. Try to talk openly with someone close about the feelings as they occur, and why you may be experiencing them. This not only creates some control over the feelings through understanding, but such sharing with a loved one can lead to deepening of trust and affection between partners.

9. *A comfortable, trusting relationship with a physician knowledgeable about MS* who is willing to deal with the varied and long-term manifestations of this chronic disease is invaluable. Many questions will arise requiring professional response. Complications can be anticipated and reduced or prevented by an alert and concerned physician. It is preferable to be involved with a doctor who works within an interdisciplinary or team setting, as various health professionals may be needed at different times. Communication between these professionals enhances and reinforces individualized care. This type of center is not available to most people, and so an appropriate "solo" practitioner is selected. This may be the family doctor, internist, or neurologist. Be sure that questions are answered satisfactorily, and follow-up appointments are scheduled. "Come back when you have a problem" often results in the recognition of problems after they have progressed needlessly.

10. *Counseling can be extremely helpful* during the period following establishment of the MS diagnosis. Although some people associate counseling or psychotherapy with mental illness or character weakness, anyone undergoing an unusual emotional stress, such as that imposed by MS, may benefit from psychological services. An objective, concerned mental health professional can help clarify feelings, goals, and choices, as well as provide valuable emotional support. Counseling may be undertaken on an individual basis for the person with MS or for a family member, a couple, or a family unit. Group counseling can be particularly helpful, as it provides an opportunity to discuss common problems and issues with others in similar circumstances. (See discussion on this subject in Chapter 12.) The interchange is maximized by the participation of a professional group leader as opposed to self-help or "rap" groups. Your physician, the local chapter of the National MS So-

ciety, or local mental health center can help define the services available in a particular community.

ONGOING PROBLEMS

Questions about interpersonal relationships persist as time goes by. One such problem involves "role expectations," or ways of behaving and reacting in situations that fit with self-image and the expectations of those around you. This includes attitudes, activities, patterns of decision-making, expressing feelings, and meeting needs of significant others. Role expectations exist in every social situation but are of greatest importance within the home and with those people with whom one is in daily or intimate contact. Some thought should be given to determine current role expectations and the ways that these might be threatened by the diagnosis of a chronic disease or by actual physical disability. A determined effort may be needed to minimize those changes that will have undesirable outcomes. Awareness of potential problem areas and pitfalls may be helpful in anticipating difficulties and bypassing disastrous outcomes.

Relationship with Parents

Look at current roles and relationships with family members, such as parents. How frequent are visits and telephone contacts with them (if not living in the same household)? During times of particular stress, such as the appearance of new symptoms or a job change, an increase in contacts can be expected. However, a general pattern of calling more often and allowing more activities to be undertaken by parents *unnecessarily* should be a warning that dependency may be growing. Given the earlier parent/child roles, it is easy for this to happen and more difficult to reverse than to prevent. It is important to be aware of the love and concern motivating parents to "do something" and to emphasize the importance of the MS person's need to maintain as much independence as possible when discussing the situation with them. Parents generally want to be helpful and appreciate honesty about how to best accomplish this. If circumstances require that more assistance be provided, relinquishing tasks or specific responsibilities to parents may be needed and greatly appreciated. Frank discussion along with accurate identification of tasks requiring assistance can facilitate the MS person's control over how help is distributed and utilized.

Parents of a young adult with MS who find themselves in the quandary of wanting to be helpful while not encouraging dependence may also find some structured reflection helpful. They may begin by considering the amount of current contact (phone calls, visits) versus that prior to diagnosis. Which of these changes reflect: (a) a need for direct care due to progressive disability; (b) relief of some activities and/or responsibilities due to progressive disability; (c) assumption of activities or responsibilities that might still be managed by the MS person? Unfortunately, certain activities may need to be relinquished by the individual, depending on the level of disability. However, the greatest favor is to assist the daughter or son to continue previous activities as much as possible. The desire to help can often be directed toward devising creative ways to make this happen: for example, suggest a telephone bill paying service, use of a device such as the Amigo to increase mobility, the use of hand controls on the car, etc. Modifications will need to be individually designed according to abilities and limitations. In those rare situations where disability is extensive, parents may find themselves assuming increasing responsibility for care without much freedom for deciding the limits. Even in such severe circumstances, choices still exist: the choice to care for the MS individual without outside help, to seek outside help from public or private agencies, to delegate care to an appropriate facility such as a health-related facility (HRF) or nursing home (skilled nursing facility or SNF). Such decisions may be best for all concerned but are usually accepted better when made with consultation of a health professional such as the physician, nurse, or social worker. Parents are not able to assume responsibility for the well-being of their child forever, particularly as MS does not often decrease life expectancy, and long-term plans must be considered.

Guilt is a common response of parents whose child has MS, possibly because of earlier roles of parental responsibility. Realistically, parents and others have no control over precipitating the onset of MS. This knowledge may not diminish the pain of such feelings, however, and professional counseling might be indicated to help parents relieve these and other painful and confusing responses.

Not all parents experience the desire to be helpful as the primary reaction. Anger, depression, and rejection may be prolonged emotional responses. In these cases, the parent's life situation may make assuming responsibility for the MS person totally unrealistic or undesirable. As stated previously, feelings are neither "good" nor "bad" in a moral sense. The parent who has struggled for many years to achieve an independent life style or retired people who at last are experiencing long-planned freedom are examples of parents who may very appropriately fear having a disabled son or daughter increasingly dependent on them. In most cases, additional physical and/or fiscal responsibility is not relegated to parents, as most people with MS do not become severely disabled. The fear and dread of this possibility, however, is very real. Acceptance of such responses by the parents themselves, the MS person, and others involved with the family can clear the way for an ongoing open and mutually supportive relationship.

Parent–child relationships are complicated in the best of circumstances, and MS only increases the confusion. It is important to remember that all involved are entitled to feel angry, depressed, and resentful. Awareness of the source of these feelings and open communication between family members help bring these painful feelings into proper perspective and increase the intimacy and support already present.

Relationship with Children

This discussion refers to preschool and school-age children, as these children are living at home and are directly affected by MS in the household. The MS parent and spouse with young or teenage children face many decisions about how to deal with MS within the family unit. Unfortunately, parents may underestimate their children and believe that denial will effectively cover up the problems of MS. These parents unwittingly communicate their worry, anxiety, and distress while trying to assure the child that everything is fine. The perceptive child may outwardly react to the verbal statements while harboring fearful fantasies. Deception about such a vital area as a parent's health implies that the truth is devastating or "unspeakable." The child may then exhibit acceptance because he has received the message that speaking openly about this topic is prohibited. The loneliness and fright the child conceals, however, may be acted out in other ways because such feelings are not easily contained. Academic difficulties, fights with classmates, truancy, withdrawal, and even delinquency can be emotional outlets for these painful feelings. These events certainly occur in the absence of MS but are more likely when the family has closed off the possibility of sharing problems openly.

The goal is not to tell children elaborate details of symptoms and potential complications. The kind of information communicated depends on the child's age, his or her ability to comprehend, and the questions asked. Appropriate articles can be given to teenagers if interest is expressed.

Advocating openness with children is not meant to imply that this will prevent or solve all potential problems surrounding the parent's MS. Should disability develop, the child's adjustment to living in a family with chronic illness can be especially difficult. Children will also be affected by the uncertainty and fluctuation of symptoms, as is the parent with MS and other close family members. The younger child's unsophisticated level of verbal communication and limited life experience occasionally create a situation best alleviated by professional counseling. A need for such counseling does not reflect inadequacies of the parents. Rather, it reflects the confusing and bewildering impact of chronic disease in the family superimposed on the normally difficult developmental tasks of growing up. Professionals who are trained in eliciting information from children are invaluable. Usually only several sessions will be needed to clarify problem areas and assist parents and child to choose effective ways of handling them.

Relationship with the Spouse

There is often a parallel between the MS person's response to chronic illness and the spouse's response. For example, the couple tends to either pursue the same patterns of socialization which existed prior to the illness or to isolate themselves from former social relationships. This dichotomy refers primarily to MS in which disability is apparent or activities are limited by easy fatigability. When isolation is chosen as the predominant pattern, it is usually a result of a reduction in the family's free time due to management of the impairment and, more significantly, to negative attitudes attributed to people outside the family. It appears that the preconception of people's reaction to physical limitation is more powerful than actual experiences. This suggests that the attitudes of the couple (more than the degree of disability) limit socialization with others. The couple need to examine their own earlier attitudes toward people with physical limitations and the resultant influence on current interpretation of other people's responses. It is also important to consider that people respond to behavior, so that the couple who convey discomfort and awkwardness elicit a similar response. Lacking awareness of this phenomenon, the couple may attribute all negative reactions to the disability. As stated earlier, such a simplified explanation is not intended to minimize the difficult adjustments that may be needed but to provide a basis for understanding and a direction for growth.

The couple's relationship with each other is also directly affected by the MS of one partner. Open communication is the basis for adjustment, assuming the pre-existence of love and trust between the spouses. The stress of a chronic illness can heighten previous interpersonal conflicts, so that positive factors need to be emphasized. Both partners will experience feelings such as anger, despair, loneliness, and self-pity—all very appropriate to the current situation. If these feelings can be shared, the sense of aloneness can be reduced. An effort by each spouse to understand the other's feelings may not only strengthen the relationship but provide an atmosphere conducive to problem solving and defining mutual goals. Adjustments must be made by both partners, a process which may necessitate dealing with very strong emotions and allowing more separate "space" than before. For example, consider a couple who enjoyed playing tennis together and can no longer do so because of the limitations of one partner. Both are resentful, but the disability of one spouse need not be imposed on the other. The non-MS partner can continue this activity and may need encouragement to do so. The spouse with MS may become active in political groups which promote the rights of disabled individuals and also needs approval to do so. What may appear as distancing in such a relationship actually allows for more freedom to enjoy each other with little resentment. Spouses need to retain separate identities, despite areas of dependence which may be necessitated by MS.

Individuality, interdependence, and mutual love and respect can be maintained, despite the impact of MS, and should be important components of all interactions between spouses. Hopefully, these feelings will also facilitate their socialization within the community. This, fortunately, is the outcome for most couples dealing with MS.

Potential Dependency Issues (Spouses)

Potential dependence within the couple may involve emotional, physical, and/or economic aspects. *Emotional dependence* occurs when the MS partner relies almost exclusively on his or her spouse for socialization, encouragement, and attention. Outside relationships may be unnecessarily relinquished, as well as participation in family decision making. *Physical dependence* includes reliance by the MS partner on his or her spouse for assistance with personal activities, such as bathing, dressing, and housekeeping or household maintenance tasks. *Economic dependence* results from diminished or lost income by the MS partner, thereby increasing the need for financial support from the non-MS spouse.

As these transitions occur, the MS person may experience feelings of frustration and a loss or reduction of the sense of self-worth. The spouse is likely also to have some negative reactions, including resentment and fear of losing a separate identity. One phenomenon which couples have described illustrates the change in patterns of relating to each other: In certain circumstances the nondisabled spouse serves as a physical or even mechanical extension of the MS person. The healthy spouse becomes the "legs," "hands," a retrieval device, or a messenger for the MS spouse. It is not the actual performance of tasks that is at issue, as these can be requested and carried out within the context of loving and caring communication. The negative interaction involves depersonalization of the nondisabled spouse, wherein commands replace requests. For the MS partner this is probably an expression of intolerable frustration, but it needs to be discussed openly if increasing resentment by the non-MS partner is to be avoided.

Emotional dependence can be eased by continued socialization with friends, both as a couple and as individuals. As noted previously, socialization is more limited by the couple's attitudes than by physical impediments, so the initiative to continue a social life must come from the couple. The disabled person can maintain friendships by telephone when get-togethers are not feasible. Both partners have a responsibility to themselves and to each other to continue valued personal and mutual friendships. This is important for each partner's self-image and enjoyment of life as well as for the health of the couple's relationship.

Another factor in preventing dysfunctional emotional dependency of one spouse is cultivation of an environment in which interdependence and mutual respect may develop or continue. The need for understanding, love, and encouragement is basic for most people, and can be shared and exchanged despite physical limitations.

Physical dependence may develop because of specific MS impairments from weakness or decreased energy, or as the result of psychological or attitudinal factors. Psychological factors include depression, "putting off" efforts while waiting for a remission, or the partner's desire to make life easier by taking on tasks rather than watch his or her spouse struggle to learn adaptive skills. These and other responses are counterproductive and need to be dealt with if physical dependence is to be kept within the boundaries of necessity.

Special problems arise when role reversal is encountered. This entails one or both spouses assuming tasks or responsibilities previously within the other partner's domain. The man whose wife has physical limitations from MS may need to take on unfamiliar child-care and housekeeping activities. The woman whose spouse becomes disabled may be confronted with household repairs, financial management, and perhaps economic support. These examples reflect traditional roles in our society and do not apply to every couple. Difficulties cannot be avoided in such circumstances, but frustration can often be eased and resentment minimized. Attitudes about male–female roles need to be flexible and tasks reassigned or "swapped" according to the family needs and the abilities of both spouses. The homemaker who must switch to wage-earner will appreciate whatever help is possible in household management from the home-bound partner. Unnecessary dependence occurs when this help does not materialize, and the MS spouse withdraws from all responsibilities. Even the severely disabled individual can perform such tasks as compiling grocery lists and calling in orders to local stores for home delivery (special telephone devices are available for the disabled, as well as operator-transmitted calls). Too often, effort is not expended by the disabled spouse to find creative ways of performing tasks or assuming new responsibilities. It is this apathy that can heighten interpersonal tension to the breaking point. Working together, at each partner's maximal level of functioning, helps maintain a positive and caring relationship.

Economic dependence resulting from decreased income, compounded by mounting medical expenses, can be the source of severe interpersonal conflict. This corresponds with couples who do not have to deal with chronic illness, where financial problems are often the core of marital conflict. Some measures can be taken to reduce this high-risk problem area. The first and crucial step is to be sure that maximal health-care insurance is in effect for the MS partner and family. The increased cost of premiums for such coverage is worth the added expense. Policies should be checked to verify coverage in the following areas: outpatient medical visits and procedures, outpatient and hospital rehabilitation, general hospital care and extended hospitalization, psychotherapy, home-care services, medications, supplies and equipment. Depletion of financial resources may be avoided by this precaution, as medical expenses in chronic illness may become astronomical.

Consideration should also be given to benefit programs, such as disability available through work and/or state and federal programs. These resources may be tapped under certain circumstances, thereby preserving personal assets. Consultation with a trusted and knowledgeable lawyer or accountant may clarify measures which will ensure continued financial stability and family security (such as trust funds for the children or mortgage-disability insurance plans).

Another important concept is continued employment, when the MS spouse is a wage-earner. Apart from valuable effects such as maintenance of self-esteem and work socialization, the continuing income is certainly an asset. Related vocational/occupational issues are addressed in Chapter 14.

SUMMARY

The unpredictable and sometimes progressive course of MS undoubtedly presents a variety of problems. However, the MS person and family can do a great deal to develop satisfactory patterns for coping with the ongoing stresses. Assistance from health professionals may give needed direction and support for strategies of adaptation. Armed with accurate information and professional guidance when needed, the MS individual and family can determine the most appropriate measures to achieve optimal function and quality of life.

14

Vocational Issues

Nancy J. Holland, Lola Sprinzeles, and Seymour R. Kaplan

For many people, positive feelings about themselves are at least partially related to job or career roles. The diagnosis of a chronic disease such as MS always threatens the individual's self-image but has a much greater impact when work activity is affected. Every effort should be made to maintain the individual's confidence and prior level of function. The potential work dropout may be facing considerable physical limitations or, responding to depression, anticipation of disability or adoption of the sick role. Whether the cause is physical or emotional, the process requires interruption at this point. It is more difficult to resume employment status than to maintain it; regaining self-esteem presents a far greater obstacle than retaining it. Although unemployment may accrue financial benefits, it can have profound repercussions: The handicapped identity is assumed, expectations of career advancement are canceled, and dependence on the government for financial support is established.

It might be helpful at this point to differentiate between some commonly used terms which may seem interchangeable but which have subtle and significant differences:

Impairment refers to the physical defect due to MS lesions with resultant loss of normal bodily mechanical function.

Disablement refers to the consequences of impairment with a reduction in functional ability.

Handicap refers to the effects of impairment or disability on the person's interactions with others and the ability to keep a satisfactory place in the community.

To illustrate these definitions, consider a person with severe visual deficiency. The actual limitation in vision is an *impairment*. When the visual problem interferes with function, such as reading or writing checks, it becomes a *disability*. When this individual applies for a job as a taxi driver or engraver, the visual deficiency is a *handicap*.

According to this terminology, measures can be taken to prevent some impairments from being disabilities. In the case mentioned, eyeglasses or a magnifier might suffice. Likewise, some handicaps can be avoided. The visually impaired person might work as a consumer advocate or insurance agent and not encounter a vocational handicap.

These distinctions are not merely semantic exercises but are intended to convey a philosophy. The impairment, or physical limitation, is usually a factor over which the individual has little control. Some choices do exist, however, as to the extent that impairment becomes a disability or handicap. These choices are particularly evident in the area of vocational adaptation.

VOCATIONAL ASSESSMENT

Changes in physical status may necessitate a reassessment of abilities and limitations relative to work requirements. As intellect is rarely impaired, remaining skills can be redirected and utilized. Even when a career change is not indicated, certain modifications may be helpful. Professional guidance and assistance with vocational problems are available through various agencies, such as the State Office or Division of Vocational Rehabilitation (OVR or DVR). Individuals with vocational or educational difficulties may look into these possibilities themselves or they may be referred by a physician or other health practitioner.

HISTORY OF VOCATIONAL EFFECTS AND CURRENT LEGISLATION

From the earliest days of our country, criteria for an acceptable life style were based on the Puritan work ethic. Poverty was attributed to an unwillingness to work. During the 1850s, in the wake of the Industrial Revolution, rapid sociological changes included transformation from rural to urban society, advanced technology, and improved life-saving measures. One outcome of these changes was increased longevity and a rise in the number of disabled persons. This population was swelled by the return of World War II disabled veterans, emphasizing the need for meaningful rehabilitation services. The current disabled population in the United States numbers about 30 million, of whom about 130,000 suffer from MS. The disabled comprise a large block of the voting constituency which is not easily ignored. This factor is reflected in social legislation such as Social Security Unemployment Insurance, Workmen's Compensation, Affirmative Action, etc. (See Chapter 16 for more detailed information.) Also, the disabled have demanded and achieved greater access to vocational pursuits.

Of particular interest to the MS person is the 1977 agreement between representatives of private and public sectors to increase and improve vocational services for the MS population. The involved agencies included:

1. Rehabilitation Services Administration (RSA, a federal agency)

2. National Multiple Sclerosis Society (NMSS, a private foundation which promotes and supports research and services related to MS)

3. Council of State Administrators of Vocational Rehabilitation (CSAVR, those state programs designed to help the disabled retain or regain productive employment)

Emphasis on extending services to the severely handicapped may also benefit those individuals who have severe disability from MS.

For those individuals who are work-ready, the Rehabilitation Act of 1973 contains useful information. This act requires that employers holding federal contracts for $2,500 or more take affirmative action to hire the disabled, and it prohibits discrimination against the disabled in promotion practices. This mandate encompasses approximately half of the businesses in America. The 1973 act also directs the employer to make "reasonable accommodations" for the handicapped employee. This includes making facilities more accessible (such as restrooms, equipment, and work areas) by installing ramps and other adaptations.

State and federal programs such as Medicaid (New York State) and Medicare provide financial assistance for medical expenses to people with disabilities. These health-care plans can assist the MS person indefinitely or until vocational goals are realized.

Another regulation aimed at effecting changes in hiring practices is the Targeted Jobs Tax Credit (TJTC). When filing federal tax returns, eligible employers claim credit for workers hired during the preceding year who received Social Security Disability Supplementary Income or who were referred by OVR or other certified placement agencies.

A provision of the Workers' Compensation Law is intended to remove deterrents from hiring disabled but occupationally qualified workers. The employer is released from the increased liability for job-related accidents which compound pre-existing disability, known by the employer at time of hiring.

Another legislative asset is continued Social Security Disability Benefits for 9 months following remunerative employment. Also, the 1980 Social Security Amendments allow for continued coverage under Medicare and Medicaid when employment cancels Social Security benefits.

VOCATIONAL REHABILITATION AGENCIES

Various agencies are concerned with providing social and vocational servies for people with disability. Agencies vary from community to community, although those which are federally administered are fairly consistent, such as the state OVR or DVR. Eligibility for services from OVR or DVR is based on residence within the particular state and existence of a handicapping physical or psychological disability. When the handicap includes severe visual impairment, the Commission for the Blind and Visually Handicapped (CBVH) is the appropriate federal agency for vocational services. Requirements include visual acuity of 20/200 (with best correction in the better eye) or limited peripheral vision of 20 degrees or less. These impairments are classified as "legal blindness," although some functional vision is often present. For the MS person, varying degrees of visual disturbance may occur. However, these generally remit and very rarely progress to legal blindness necessitating intervention by CBVH. Assistance that both of the above agencies offers includes financial support of educational effort, retraining programs, adaptive devices such as a typewriter or automobile hand controls, essential medical evaluations, and transportation costs during the period of sponsorship. Ongoing counseling programs, job-related tools, and mobility aids may also be subsidized. According to individual needs, job placement and help with post-employment problems (that is, follow-up services) are provided. It should be emphasized that many individuals who are no longer capable of functioning in their established work area can be retrained to be productive and self-supporting in other areas.

Despite the many adversities of MS there are some encouraging features. The life span is relatively unaffected, intellect is rarely impaired, and the usually long remission periods can be effectively utilized for occupational pursuits. Although there is no cure for the disease, many disabling symptoms can be effectively treated, and the majority of those individuals diagnosed never experience severe disability.

POSSIBLE ADAPTIVE MEASURES

There are many potential alterations the person with MS can consider in order to keep or secure a job. Choices depend on the individual's difficulties and needs, work environment and job description, imagination, and determination. The following are representative options for consideration, as well as ideas to stimulate the development of other adaptive measures.

1. Fluctuating energy levels may be circumvented by work which is task-oriented rather than time-oriented, has intermittent or staggered work hours, or allows lunch time naps; self-employment and homebound work on consignment are also possibilities.

2. Physical limitations may be overcome by shifting from a physically demanding job to a sedentary one. Consider transfer to a different department within the firm or relocation to another branch

of the company where appropriate positions are available or architectural barriers are absent.

3. Commuting difficulties can be minimized by employment within a more geographically accessible area. A desirable locale might be one along a negotiable bus route or within a financially reasonable taxi zone. Private taxi companies may provide assistance with appliances such as a walker or wheelchair for regular customers. Participation in a car pool is also a possibility.

4. Adaptive devices can compensate for some physical impairments. Some examples:

a. Automobile hand controls when driving ability is affected by leg weakness or incoordination.

b. Voice amplification devices when weak vocal projection is a problem.

c. Optical aids to offset some visual impairments.

d. Calculators, electric typewriters, and remote control units to compensate for upper extremity involvement.

e. Assistance devices for ambulation, such as a cane or walker, to afford greater mobility and help prevent falls.

f. Motorized "scooters," such as the Amigo and Portascoot, when mobility or easy fatigability is a problem.

In addition to hand controls, procurement of a "disabled driver's parking permit" increases access by automobile. Also, a citizen-band transmitter/receiver installed in the car can be utilized to summon assistance during an emergency. For the disabled driver, even a flat tire may produce a crisis situation if help is not near by.

For those using public transportation, the cost can be reduced by the "Half-Fare Program for the Handicapped" available in most communities.

More ideas for adaptive measures to directly or indirectly support occupational efforts can be found in Chapter 8.

COUNSELING PROGRAMS

Living with chronic disease imposes enormous stress on the MS person and family. The strain may be evident in the interpersonal relationships within the family, as well as in social and work interactions outside the home. Adaptation to such pervasive stress may be eased by involvement in a counseling program that can provide information, objectivity, understanding, and emotional support. Many counseling formats are available. The individual, couple, or family may relate to a therapist alone or may be involved in a group situation with other MS individuals, couples, or families led by a therapist or co-therapies. Some therapies are time-limited and last for a specified time frame (such as 1 hour a week for 10 sessions), whereas others are ongoing, without a definite termination point. Counseling may also be focused on a particular issue, such as vocational or occupational problems.

Self-help groups are specifically information/emotional support-oriented and, although helpful, should not be confused with professional counseling. Self-help groups cannot provide the objectivity and skills a professional therapist contributes, and they lack accountability to clients and do not assume responsibility for the participants' protection and growth.

The type of counseling program selected depends on: (a) available services within the community; (b) the needs and problems of the MS person, couple, spouse, or other family member; (c) the desire and motivation for assistance; and (d) the financial resources of the client relative to cost of various therapies. It is important to note that people who would not seek counseling under normal conditions may benefit greatly from such services given the unusual stress of a chronic illness such as MS.

Special mention should be made of the growing recognition of the group format as a method of improving social and vocational adaptation of MS individuals and families. Such groups range from lecture/discussion sessions to professionally led psychotherapy groups, as previously mentioned. A common feature of all types is the unifying experience that reduces the person's sense of isolation with the disease.

Objectives of Group Intervention

The overall objective of group intervention is to improve interpersonal growth through education, shared experiences, and discussion of dependency issues.

Education: It has been demonstrated that some people are better able to accept the diagnosis of MS if they understand the nature of the illness and the specific complications from which they suffer (such as disturbances of gait, visual problems, fatigue, sexual dysfunction, bladder/bowel incontinence). For many, however, the ability to understand (to "hear") depends on receiving emotional support in order to accept the implications of this serious physical disorder. The group situation can help provide that needed emotional support.

Shared experiences: The shared MS experience is conducive to the development of trust. The similarity of problems encountered in the daily experience of individuals with MS can become the basis of discussion and lead to the exploration of coping techniques within an accepting and empathetic environment.

Discussion of dependency issues: There are many factors that generate anger in the MS person: the realistic helplessness imposed by physical limitations, the fear of progressive physical deterioration, the turmoil that inevitably is expressed by the question "Why me?," the changed function in social roles (parent, spouse, worker). The emotional bond among group members and the supportive role of the group leaders make it possible for the counselees to turn the feelings of dependency into a constructive effort in order to achieve a greater sense of control over one's life and more effective means of coping with the various stresses of MS.

SUMMARY

Working provides an important source of self-esteem and financial independence for many people, including those with MS. Maintenance of employment is more easily achieved than re-employment, and so every effort should be made to continue work activities, with whatever modifications are needed. Assistance is available for those who desire vocational guidance, and many options are possible for people with MS desirous of gainful employment.

15

What About New Treatments?

Robert J. Slater

There are many reasons why the MS person in today's world is frequently confused, frustrated, and even cynical about what and whom to believe about treatments and claims for improvement in their symptoms. Our advances in research have not yet pinpointed the basic errors in function causing the autoimmune reaction that may produce MS. Consequently, it has not been possible to produce specific drugs or vaccines to prevent or cure MS, or even to predictably decrease the severity in different stages of the illness. As in the case with other chronic illnesses caused by autoimmune reactions (for instance, rheumatoid arthritis, lupus, certain types of diabetes, and myasthenia gravis), only a breakthrough in research will focus on what is wrong and what specific treatment is necessary. It is well to remember, though, that such breakthroughs have been made over the past 50 years: for instance, virus vaccines to prevent polio, measles, and other childhood virus infections; penicillin and other antibiotics to eradicate bacterial infections; insulin to control diabetes; L-DOPA for Parkinson's disease.

At this time, scientists and clinicians are excited about how much new information is arising from advances in research and the technological wonders that increase the sensitivity of research that will provide a similar control of MS. So there is good reason to have faith that we are much closer to some answers. Much new and detailed information about the planets has been made possible during the past decade by the invention of space probes, and the same tremendous advances are occuring from biological probes that map normal and abnormal activity in the cells and tissues of our bodies.

In the meantime, we are faced with the age-old problem that when there is no specific treatment all sorts of fads and claims for success are promoted. Not only patients but frequently physicians have difficulty sorting out fact from fancy.

FACTORS INFLUENCING THE PATIENT'S RESPONSE

In order to grasp what is involved in judging what to do until we find a specific treatment, there are a number of important factors to consider. First, there is the problem of interpreting the natural clinical course of relapses and remissions in many MS persons—the bouts of worsening followed by spontaneous improvement. Such cyclical change is absolutely unpredictable and varies in degree from person to person. For example, if one has just started a new dietary treatment and improvement occurs, we want to know if it was caused by the treatment or if it is a spontaneous remission. Because of the variation in timing and severity of MS bouts from one patient to another, it is usually impossible to measure specific improvement in less than at least 2 years.

The second factor in understanding how our bodies respond in MS is the marvelous power of the body for self-healing. This power is augmented by faith that a particular treatment will help. This is called the placebo response. Because of the strong influence of our personality and behavior on how our bodies function, for better or worse, the placebo response can mimic a positive response to treatment in a high percentage of people, perhaps half or more.

Again the same question can be asked. What if one has started a new dietary treatment and improvement in feeling and function occurs—was the improvement caused by our inherent behavioral response toward self-healing? If so, then it was a placebo response and not specifically induced by the treatment.

A third factor in understanding the effect of treatment is the likelihood of placebo responsiveness of the body at different stages of MS. In early relapsing and remitting illness, with or without gradual accumulation of handicaps, there is believed to be a greater potential for placebo response to occur and confuse the interpretation of the effect of a treatment being tried. In later, chronic-progressive or chronic-stable MS, the placebo response may be present but is believed to have a lesser effect. It is important for MS persons to remember that doctors, when testing a treatment, cannot distinguish improvement due to a placebo response from a specific healing effect of a treatment form without a carefully controlled clinical study.

THE PLACEBO RESPONSE

Much importance is attached to the natural healing power of the body, the placebo response, and what regulates these behavioral reactions, and so a great deal of research is directed to this field. What has become clear is that any situation which increases the belief or faith of a person that some action will lead to a favorable outcome enhances the likelihood that at least some alleviation of symptoms will occur and will last for a while. These situations include the faith of the patient in the doctor, or any other healer, as well as religious faith. Such responses are often augmented when these experiences of faith and hope are shared by others in a group. The favorable response to belief and faith are clearly part of the doctor–patient relationship, an outcome of a shared experience by attendance at a treatment center, and by religious faith and or visitation to a shrine. Having some form of faith is a very important part of maintaining a positive and hopeful outlook on life. The behavioral responses set in motion are increasingly understood to be associated with stress reduction. Norman Cousins noted the powerful effect of faith in the partnership with his physician, and how self-determination to reduce worry and stress by positive thinking resulted in a profound healing effect.

Understanding that stress can be harmful, leading to damage of the cardiovascular and other systems, is an important indicator of finding ways to reduce stress of MS problems on a day-to-day basis. Research has indicated that these behavioral variations that result from stress are probably mediated by hormones produced in the brain that regulate responses of the nervous system, heart and blood vessels, digestion, etc. Learning how to reduce stress and, by association, to optimize an ongoing placebo response are important factors in coping with MS.

Emphasis is directed at stress reduction by such behavioral modifiers as faith and belief and its relation to the placebo response because of the tremendous importance in interpreting the results of treatment. In view of the above understandings, it is apparent that the placebo response is a normal psychosomatic reaction that can influence the course of an apparent illness; the response varies from person to person and to some extent in the same person from time to time. It is also important to remember that the symptoms caused by the areas of MS inflammation can have superimposed symptoms induced by stress and a psychosomatic response. Thus when a patient undergoes the stress-reducing placebo response, the disappearance of psychosomatic symptoms of disability is interpreted as clinical improvement, albeit the primary MS symptoms remain unchanged. Because of the great variation in personalities and behavioral responses among people, some MS individuals may have relatively minor neurological disability but a major psychosomatic extension of those symptoms. In such a person a placebo response would have a marked effect. Another MS person may have much more severe disability with little or no stress-induced psychosomatic overlay. In this person, little or no placebo-induced improvement would be expected.

The implications of these normal behavioral responses which effect us all are important in assessing both the patient's and the physician's approach to unproved therapies or clinical trials. Four factors which influence behavior in individuals have been noted:

1. Persons with any chronic illness are psychologically vulnerable and may become desperate and grasp at therapeutic straws so that emotions rather than common sense determine their decisions.

2. Many people are strongly suggestible so that even without new areas of MS inflammation unconscious anxiety may now be expressed as MS-like symptoms, such as numbness or weakness. These symptoms can be reversed by reassurance and persuasion from a physician (stress reduction) but likewise may be reversed by belief in a new therapeutic caprice (placebo response).

3. The practice of medicine based on ideals of service and sound scientific principles may be usurped by the business of medical

practice in which remedies are offered indiscriminately. Here again uncritical belief by a patient and suggestibility may lead to temporary reversal of symptoms that results from the placebo response.

4. Sincere doctors themselves may be the victims of suggestibility and, given the concurrence of a clinical improvement associated with some form of therapy, may interpret the cause/effect response uncritically, even to the point, in some instances, of developing a messiah attitude.

Therefore the dilemma faced by patients and their physicians is that, given the confusing picture caused by the natural tendency for remissions, as well as the placebo response, and also given the fact that there is no predictable treatment—what is there to do? One can argue that the principle "It can't hurt; it might help; let's try it" be invoked, but that denies scientific integrity. This problem is compounded by the situation that numerous therapeutic trials have been conducted by clinicians of impeccable qualifications on the basis of leads from scientific research. The fact that over the years none of these has proved any more successful than the most unscientific remedy has made it difficult to say that one form of therapy is any better than another.

Given this wide range of circumstances which must be considered in day-to-day care, the National Multiple Sclerosis Society has supported the decision of physicians who recommend unproved therapies (such as diets or vitamin supplements), provided the therapy has no record of harmful response and that the treatment will not compromise the financial integrity of the patient because of high professional fees, interruption in employment, costs of travel, and living at a distant location. It is imperative that any such trials be conducted with the ongoing support of the personal physician so that he remains identified with the patient's overall care.

THE ROLE OF CLINICAL TRIALS

Because it is so difficult to determine when a treatment is truly effective and predictable in a way that distinguishes it from the results obtained with a placebo or spontaneous remission, three outcomes may be used to determine the effectiveness of a treatment.

1. A completely effective agent would be relatively simple to recognize because it would prevent relapses and halt progression in all stages of the disease.

2. An entirely ineffective or placebo agent would be associated with a significant rate of improvement especially in the early stages of MS.

3. A partially effective agent would be difficult to recognize because of the placebo/remission situation and would require study under controlled conditions.

With advances in research pointing to the potential value of treatments that involve correction of the adverse autoimmune response, increasing emphasis is being placed on trials of new drugs. Similarly, when a claim to improvement is made for some form of treatment, such as a specific diet, then controlled scientific studies are required to determine the veracity of the claim.

Two forms of clinical trial are used to test the efficacy of a treatment. For a beginning, a *preliminary trial* on a few patients provides a reflection of possible toxic side effects and an understanding of the dosage required. Afterward, a *longitudinal trial* is conducted that involves groups of patients in various stages of MS followed for 2 years or more. This length of time is necessary because of the relative infrequency and unpredictability of naturally occurring relapses or the rate of worsening of slowly progressive MS. Because of the placebo response, only if the therapy is associated with cessation of progress in the disease or marked diminution of the relapse rate in 90 to 100% of cases can it be said to be effective. This high level of success is required to distinguish it from the placebo response. Intermediate responses could be expected from a partially effective agent and would be difficult to interpret.

A *double-blind matched randomized controlled trial* is used to confirm preliminary results from a longitudinal trial. In this situation, patients must consent to participate in the trial because they will be allocated randomly to one of two groups—one to receive the medication under trial and the other to receive a blank, or placebo. Double-blind means that not only do the patients not know whether they are receiving the drug or a placebo, neither do the doctors. The materials are given with code numbers, and a confidential list of allocations is maintained by a responsible third party until the study ends or in case the trial is stopped because of adverse reactions. Such a trial also may require 2 to 3 years of observation, but it is the only method to differentiate the placebo response.

The importance of the double-blind technique was emphasized in the 1968 study of ACTH treatment in early relapsing/remitting MS that was conducted collaboratively in 10 university medical centers. After 1 month of therapy, 70% of patients on placebo had a clinical improvement comparable to that achieved in the ACTH group. This result reflected the placebo effect plus the natural remission effect and threw great doubt on the clinical effectiveness of ACTH. Current thinking is that ACTH or steroids may lessen the severity of a relapse but have no influence on the long-term course of MS.

THE CONTINUING PANOPLY OF THERAPEUTIC CLAIMS

Down through the years, since MS was first described by Charcot in 1864, over 100 different treatments have been tried. None have stood the test of time, but recent advances in immunosuppressive therapy hold promise for slowing or halting the progress of the disease.

Three significant points require emphasis when interpreting clinical anecdotes or deciding to undertake another form of therapy:

1. No treatment of any kind has yet proved to have a predictable and specific response in interrupting the basic disease process which causes MS.

2. A number of therapies are helpful in ameliorating some of the symptoms of MS and are universally prescribed (drugs for the treatment of spasticity, imbalance in the control of bladder and bowel, mental depression, and pain).

3. Therapeutic trials and treatments are encouraged by three groups of professionals: (a) scientists studying the basic disease process of MS who judge that some new biological evidence may prove helpful in interrupting the course of the disease; (b) sincere physicians in

practice who hold well-meaning beliefs in certain current hypotheses about the disease process of MS or whose belief that certain therapeutic claims may help their patients; and (c) a variety of professionals, therapists, and cultists who respond to the large population of individuals with chronic illness by offering various nostrums and manipulations or combinations of formulations in a manner that, while outwardly displaying a patina of professional competence, in fact are preying on the psychological vulnerability of the patient.

A classification of modern therapies for MS has been published by the National Multiple Sclerosis Society in which the following categories are outlined and a brief description of the treatments and what is known about their effectiveness is described. Some treatment forms are based on theories of the cause of MS, some on ideas about the mode of its development, some on symptoms of the disease which might be relieved, and finally a miscellaneous or empirical group for many of which there may be no rational basis.

A few of these treatments are noted briefly here in order to emphasize the wide range of approaches and to reiterate that when no specific treatment has been developed a variety of trial-and-error efforts is bound to continue.

1. Nutrition
   a. Diets
   b. Vitamins, minerals, other nutrients
      Note: There is no evidence that any nutritional element or diet will predictably alter the course of MS.

2. Metabolic systems
   a. Carbohydrate
   b. Fat
   c. Miscellaneous
      Note: Although these basic elements of diet and of body physiological processes may be involved in inflammation, the immune response, etc., there is no scientific evidence that their metabolism can be altered in any way influencing the course of MS.

3. Vascular system
   a. Anticoagulant agents
   b. Vasodilator agents
   c. Circulatory stimulants
   Note: No efforts to influence vascular dynamics have shown any effect on the course of MS.

4. Inflammation
   a. ACTH and adrenal corticosteroids—used widely to diminish the severity of relapse in MS
   b. Protease inhibitors
   c. Agents affecting prostaglandin pathways
   d. Miscellaneous anti-inflammatory agents
   Note: A number of agents are under study to determine potential to inhibit the severity of MS inflammation and its effect on neural conduction.

5. Immune system
   a. Immunosuppression
   b. Immunomodulation
   c. Desensitization or specific immune tolerance
   Note: This area represents the most active arena of research and clinical trials because of the known abnormalities of the immune regulation in MS.

6. Infective cause
   a. Antiviral chemotherapy
   b. Vaccines and antisera
   c. Interferon and interferon inducers
   Note: Clinical trials are under way with antiviral drugs and interferons but are difficult to control because of the complexity of the materials.

7. Symptomatic treatments
   a. Affecting conduction
   b. Affecting spasticity
   c. Affecting mood, behavior motivation
   d. Physical medicine

8. Miscellaneous empirical treatments
    a. Injected materials
    b. Physical and surgical manipulations

9. Combined regimens
    a. Spas/"clinics"

Based on the best scientific projections, two lines of treatment seem to hold the greatest promise for turning off the disease process. The first is antiviral chemotherapy based on the theory that MS may be caused by one or more viruses. A longer-term projection would be that a viral vaccine for preventive immunization may be developed.

Depression or alteration of the abnormal immune response is the second line of approach. Current therapies under trial have a major impact on body function associated with many undesirable toxic side effects but show promise of slowing the natural course of MS. Future projections look to highly targeted, "magic bullet" drugs or biological agents that can specifically interrupt the abnormal immune process.

Anti-inflammatory agents are under study which will more specifically diminish the degree of inflammatory response of MS which causes the demyelination and the interruption in neural circuitry. However, such agents do not interrupt the causative process of the disease. Symptomatic treatments to reduce the effects of spasticity, pain, depression, bladder and bowel muscular imbalance, and fatigue will continue to be investigated and undoubtedly will improve maintenance of body function pending breakthrough of an agent to halt or reverse the disease.

In our current era, the rapid acceleration in research and technological information is aimed sharply at the fundamental facts of biological life that have gone wrong to result in MS. Reinforcement of our natural behavioral propensity to heal must be maintained through the belief that we can cope with the disease and that a specific treatment eventually will be found.

16

Available Services

Diann Geronemus and Leon Zitzer

Care for MS patients is complex and presents ongoing problems for the patient, family, health care providers, and community. Needs for care are unpredictable and vary greatly, given the differing presentations, symptoms, and levels of disability found in MS. The illness itself poses difficult diagnostic and management dilemmas. Some MS problems are common to other chronic disabilities as well.

Regardless of the severity of the physical and psychological impairment, some type of care is required in the following areas: (a) pharmacologic intervention; (b) medical and vocational rehabilitation; (c) bladder and bowel therapy; (d) counseling for psychological and sexual adaptation; (e) modification of the home and work environment; (f) special adaptations for transportation, recreation, and other activities of daily living; and (g) advice on economic management. Ideally, the system of human services within which care is given is responsive to the unique problems confronting MS patients and families as well as those problems MS persons share with other persons suffering from chronic illnesses.

Previous chapters have discussed care for MS patients in the areas of pharmacologic intervention; treatment with physical measures, including occupational therapy and activities of daily living; social and vocational adaptations; nursing care; bowel and bladder management; and psychological and sexual adjustments. Here these subjects are discussed insofar as they relate to a broad framework of continuing comprehensive care for MS patients and their families, and to some specific services and programs currently available under governmental and voluntary auspices.

PROVISION OF MEDICAL AND SOCIAL CARE

Short- and long-term management in MS comprises many inter-related medical and social problems. Management involves two types of professional organization: the medical model and the helping model. In the medical model the emphasis is on diagnosis and management, with care generally being rendered in a structured setting such as a hospital, clinic, or office. This type of care lends itself more readily to acute-phase, episodic problem solving. In the helping model there is an emphasis on "wellness," on helping the patient develop problem-solving techniques, and on establishing links to community-based services in order to assemble necessary psychosocial and rehabilitative services. It is within this framework that more emphasis is optimally placed on the needs of chronically ill persons and on the provision of long-term social supports for this population.

It is commonplace to hear of situations in which patients and families living with MS have been poorly handled, misdiagnosed, or, more basically, misunderstood. Unfortunately, unresponsiveness in short-term management may lead to unnecessary obstacles in the need for continuing adaptations and dynamic management in the course of a chronic illness such as MS. Barriers to effective care can occur in the medical, psychosocial, or rehabilitation spheres. For example, poor early psychological and social adaptations to changing roles and work capabilities may set up barriers to long-term patient and family adjustments, just as inadequate early evaluation of bowel and bladder symptoms can lead to embarrassing and at times life-threatening chronic medical problems.

Some basic problems have been identified which underlie the provision of services to MS patients and families. Some of these problems are inherent in the disease process itself, and others relate to the system within which needs arise and human services are developed to meet patient needs. These problems include: (a) the long-term, protracted nature of the medical and psychosocial needs; (b) unpredictability in the clinical course and severity of the disease; (c) fragmentation under different sponsorship and location of the mix of human services available to meet needs, and the wide variation of services from one community to another; (d) a lack of coherence or coordination among those fragmented services; (e) difficulty experienced by many patients in obtaining access to services; and (f) economic instability resulting from uncertain employment and income in addition to the unpredictable costs of medical and social services.

MATCHING SERVICE TO NEED

At this point it is useful to examine a model of care that matches human services to patients' needs. Any such model must take into account existing patterns of federal–state reimbursements for relevant services, the political realities of evolving institutions and laws, the values of the society in which the system exists, and the knowledge and attitudes of individuals who will influence the disabled person and family directly or indirectly. Coordination of services is the goal of such an organizational model. A conceptual framework consisting of a three-sided spectrum of resources can provide an optimal mix of services.

Governmental service departments (health, welfare, rehabilitation, etc.) are represented on one side. Community, private, and public service institutions and agencies are represented on the second side; and volunteer citizens comprise the third component. Some of this third sector operates under tax-exempt status as fund-raising agencies to provide specific services, and other volunteers function as agents of good will. Certain constraints are inherent in the development and implementation of services due to governmental regulations. Regardless, close coordination and communication within the system are essential to generate optimal services.

THE TEAM APPROACH

Within the three-sided system of services described, it is necessary to bring together a variety of professionals and lay persons who possess the knowledge and capabilities for dealing with the range of problems presented by MS patients and families. This confluence of professionals is consistent with the "team approach" to patient management. The team has increasingly been found to be effective in the provision of care to populations with long-term needs such as those found in MS. The team approach involves the physician and professionals in such disciplines as nursing; social work; clinical psychology; occupational, speech, and physical therapy; vocational rehabilitation counseling; and the clergy. The team approach can be utilized with many types of medical and psychological problems and is practiced in varied settings. The composition of the team varies depending on two factors: the setting and the patients' needs. Team efforts are directed toward providing: (a) openness of communication on behalf of the patients; (b) continuity of care; (c) a multitude of available services; (d) a stable knowledge base; (e) ongoing education about the illness and related problems; and (f) psychological as well as physical support systems.

The team can provide enormous support for the MS patient and family, beginning with the earliest symptoms, to the disclosure of a diagnosis, through the minor and major crises posed by the progression of the illness. Whenever financially and physically feasible, some combination of professionals are brought together as a team.

PROGRAMS AND SERVICES FOR THE DISABLED

Certain types of general information about programs and services are available as part of the coordinated care ideally provided by this team. This information forms an essential knowledge base for MS patients and families regardless of the type of symptomatology, the level of disability, and the system of care. A look at this informational base begins with a discussion of governmentally mandated programs for the disabled. We then consider treatment modalities for varying levels of disability in MS and finally look at services available in local communities that provide the necessary care and treatment.

Governmental Programs for the Disabled

Governmental benefits for the disabled are established by law and are subject to change. This is equally true for federal programs such as Medicare and Social Security, and for federal–state programs such as Medicaid. Additionally, federal–state programs are subject to significant variations among the states. It is helpful, however, to discuss some of the more general and stable features of these programs as they are relevant to persons with MS. Under the Social Security laws there are two separate cash benefit programs for the disabled: Social Security Disability Insurance (SSDI) and Supplemental Security Income (SSI). There are also two programs of medical assistance: Medicare and Medicaid. Eligibility criteria for these programs vary and are directly or indirectly based on meeting (a) the programs' mandated definition of disability and (b) the mandated financial requirements.

Definition of Disability

To be considered disabled under the social security law a person must have a physical or mental condition which prevents him from engaging in any substantial gainful activity (SGA) that exists in the national economy and which is expected to last (or has lasted) for at least 12 continuous months. Inability to do your regular work does not constitute disability. One must be prepared to show that he or she is unable to engage in any other type of gainful employment in order to be considered. For example, if the patient previously worked as a sales clerk but medical evidence indicates that he is capable of light sedentary work (office work) and possesses appropriate skills, it is quite likely that the claim will be denied.

The Social Security Administration maintains a medical listing for each disability category. In MS this means that one must have (a) significant and persistent disorganization of motor functions in two extremities resulting in sustained disturbance of gross and dexterous movements or of gait and station; or (b) very significant visual impairment or mental impairment. A combination of medical and vocational problems which make it extremely difficult to work may also meet the criteria. Given the great variability and unpredictability found in MS, it is the *severity* of the condition that must be documented.

A detailed report is essential to any disability claim. Good and sufficient medical evidence will show the severity of the condition as well as the extent to which it prevents the patient from undertaking substantial gainful employment. Inadequate information at the outset may necessitate a laborious appeal procedure and, at times, the involvement of legal counsel.

Two unique MS-related problems are of particular concern in disability determinations. The first relates to the date of onset of the disability and the second to the fatigue factor. Determining the date which disability began can be crucial in SSDI cases because of the length of time involved in making the diagnosis of MS during which MS patient's eligibility may have lapsed. Thus it may be critical to convince the Social Security Administration that a patient actually had MS many years before a definite diagnosis was given and that the symptoms were severe enough to cause disability at the time the patient was still insured.

Although it is often a major reason for an MS patient's inability to work, fatigue causes no outward disability and is considered a subjective symptom. This is difficult to document in disability claims. However, legally a substantially documented subjective symptom based on a verifiable medical condition such as MS may be grounds for disability. Such documentation may come from professionals or friends who have known the patient over a long period of time. This must be taken into consideration by the Social Security Administration even if at the level of a hearing.

Cash Benefit Programs—SSDI

SSDI benefits are based on the patients' work history. For workers qualifying prior to July 1980, one must have worked 20 out of the previous 40 quarters (3-month periods) before becoming disabled, essentially 5 of the previous 10 years. For workers entitled to benefits July 1980 or later, there is a more complicated, graduated scale depending on the worker's age. This work requirement poses an obstacle to eligibility in MS with its greater number of female patients as it excludes housewives who have been out of the competitive labor market for varying lengths of time. Once disability has been established, there is a 5 month waiting period until payments begin. In certain cases, retroactive payments up to 12 months may be applicable.

SSI

SSI is a public assistance benefit based on financial need rather than work history. One must meet maximum income and resource (savings, tangible assets) levels in order to qualify, as well as the disability requirements. SSDI benefits and the income of a nondisabled spouse are considered in the determination of SSI eligibility. How marital status affects income eligibility for SSI is a complicated issue and sometimes requires legal advice. States have the option of supplementing federal payments to SSI beneficiaries so that income criteria for this program varies from state to state. In certain cases where one is pursuing a vocational goal approved by the Social Security Administration and the state vocational rehabilitation agency, one may still be eligible for SSI under the self-support plan, even though income exceeds normal eligibility criteria. In such cases the cost of certain impairment related items and services (transportation, equipment) needed in the pursuit of the vocational goal can be deducted from income and resources.

Medical Assistance Programs—Medicare

Medicare is a federally funded medical insurance program. A disabled person becomes entitled to Medicare after receiving SSDI benefits for 2 years (24 months). For disabled persons under the age of 65 this is the only means to eligibility for Medicare. The program has two parts: hospital insurance (part A) and medical insurance (part B). The former can help pay for medically necessary inpatient hospital care. Under certain circumstances it also covers inpatient care in a skilled nursing facility and care in the home by an approved home health agency. Medicare medical insurance can help pay for medically necessary doctors' services; outpatient hospital, physical therapy, and speech pathology services; and some medical services, supplies, and necessary home health services not covered by the hospital insurance part of Medicare. Medicare coverage does not pay the full cost of covered services.

Medicaid

Medicaid is a federal–state medical assistance program based on financial need. Financial eligibility requirements and services provided under the program vary from state to state. In some states Medicaid and SSI eligibility are the same, and one becomes eligible for both programs simultaneously.

Some states have a surplus (excess) income program. This allows the person with an income greater than that for Medicaid eligibility, but who meets all other requirements, to obtain Medicaid coverage by spending the "excess income" on medical expenses. Medicaid will then pay for medical expenses incurred. Medicaid is not a substitute for national health insurance and does not allow a middle-income family to keep its income and still be eligible for the program. In some states there is also a catastrophic health insurance provision.

Home Health Services

Different types of home health services are provided under the Medicare and Medicaid program. Under the prescription of a physician, home health care services are provided under the Medicare program when the patient is homebound and requires intermittent skilled nursing, physical therapy, or speech therapy services. These include the insertion and sterile irrigation of catheters, application of dressings involving prescription medication and aseptic techniques, giving of injections, or performing physical therapy exercises. Personal care services can be provided by a home health aide in patients who require skilled nursing services. Medicare home health services do not provide what is considered custodial care (for example, feeding, bathing, transferring from bed to wheelchair). However, some of these needs may be met so long as a skilled nursing need is evident. There is no limit to the total number of home health care visits as long as the basic criteria are met. Medicare does not provide any home health services in what the program interprets as "chronic illness."

Medicaid home health care services vary widely from state to state. In some states the services and eligibility are similar to those of Medicare. In other states, provisions are broader and include some custodial care, housekeeper services for help with household chores, and homemaker services for help with shopping and preparing meals. The length of time that these services can be provided varies considerably from state to state. As an example of the wide variation, some states provide no custodial services, whereas a liberal interpretation exists in California: Home support services (personal care) are provided to working disabled persons if they once received SSI and became ineligible because of returning to work.

Work Incentives

After successfully obtaining benefits under the cash benefit and medical assistance programs outlined, it is difficult to contemplate a return to work and subsequent loss of such benefits. Recent changes in the law are more supportive of a recipient's attempt to return to the work force while protecting his or her benefits. The law allows disabled persons to test their ability to work for a 9-month trial period and subsequent 3-month adjustment period while benefits continue. Some changes added by the 1980 Social Security Amendments include: automatic re-entitlement to benefits within 12 months if one again becomes unable to work after SSDI or SSI payments stop; continuation of Medicare benefits for 3 years after SSDI benefits cease because of a return to substantial gainful employment; re-entitlement to Medicare immediately if a worker starts receiving SSDI benefits again within 5 years after they end and was previously entitled to Medicare; and under a 3-year experimental program, begun in 1981, allowing SSI recipients to return to work while continuing to receive Medicaid and social services necessary to maintain the work and cash benefits on a gradually decreasing scale.

At the time of this writing, more restrictive changes in all aspects of the Social Security laws are under consideration. One can keep up with changes in the Social Security law by contacting the Social Security Administration and by contacting local legal services. Pamphlets discussing the various programs are available through the local Social Security office (Appendix A).

Care in the Voluntary Sector

Returning to our three-sided system of services, we now consider the care provided in the other two sectors—the community caregivers and citizens' groupings. Here, too, the types and extent of services available vary greatly from area to area and are based on perceived need, available physical and financial resources, the allocation of such resources, and the communication and collaboration between and among the populations in need and the persons and organizations providing services.

Services are based on a person's illness stage. The need for help varies according to the disability and must be responsive to the problems of (a) newly diagnosed patients and their families; (b) minimally to moderately disabled patients and their families; and (c) severely disabled patients and their families or caretakers. Certain needs and the services to meet them are common to all three levels. A natural movement in treatment approaches and service needs exists from one level to another. Specific goals and tasks of the service-giver vary, as do the needs of the patient and family at any given level. It is important to note that in planning and providing any services there is a consideration of the total patient–family situation. It takes into account day-to-day needs, role relationships, values, perceptions of the consequences of the illness, vocational status, and family support systems.

Patients and families should find out about the services and resources available as early as possible. One might ask why such information should be obtained when there is no apparent problem as yet. We advocate getting complete information as early as possible in order to most expediently meet the long-term comprehensive need of MS persons and families. Knowledge about counseling programs, economic resources, equipment, and home care services can be readily accepted, less threatening, and less anxiety provoking if it is part of a total system of care. The knowledge can be integrated into long-term planning and problem solving with the goal of preventing crises or, at least, mitigating the effects of illness-related crisis situations. This becomes an educational process similar to the education about side effects of medication, bladder management, and skin care discussed in earlier chapters.

What do care and services mean for the MS patient and family? In broad groupings, these may include a range of counseling services, training programs, concrete services, and educational programs.

Counseling services include individual, group, couple, and family therapy; sexual counseling; and crisis intervention. In some areas specialized counseling services are available through MS clinical centers, MS chapter supported programs, and neurology departments in medical centers. Such programs would be oriented to the specialized needs of the MS population and would involve various members of the professional team discussed earlier in this chapter. Group counseling would include professionally led groups and self-help groups organized and led by MS patients and families. Various types of therapy are also available through community-based family service and mental health agencies; the outpatient department of hospital and clinics; and private practitioners—physicians, clinical psychologists, social workers, marriage and family counselors, and the clergy.

Though it is not always the primary reason for entering therapy, MS will always have some impact on the treatment goals of therapy and the means taken to achieve them. At times, in the course of any of the forms of counseling mentioned, information regarding the illness, specific symptoms, and management may be shared (with the patient's permission) by the person providing the primary medical care and the therapist. This enhances understanding of the effects of the illness on adjustment in other areas, increases communication, and maximizes coordination of care for the MS patient and family.

Training programs are generally made available through the local offices of the state vocational rehabilitation agencies (OVR or DVR). Though not in the voluntary sector, they should be mentioned at this point. Vocational rehabilitation services may be available even if a person does not meet the requirements for disability benefits. These may include one or more of the following: counseling and guidance to discuss problems and interests in order to work out a rehabilitation program that may lead to achieving self-support; the provision of medical, surgical, or hospital services to reduce or remove disability; physical aids such as artificial limbs, braces, eyeglasses; job training in a vocational school, college, or rehabilitation facility; and job placement and follow-up.

Increasing numbers of MS patients throughout the country have become involved in state vocational rehabilitation programs since 1978 as a result of a joint agreement entered into by the National Multiple Sclerosis Society, the Rehabilitation Services Administration, and the Council of State Administrators of Vocational Rehabilitation. The purposes of the agreement were to work toward more effective coordination of these agencies' resources in order to increase education, promote early identification and referral of persons in need of rehabilitation, improve service techniques to MS persons, and increase the number of MS persons having gainful employment. Progress has been made in this area, though specific program activity varies from state to state. Some hospitals and rehabilitation centers offer limited vocational training, usually in a sheltered workshop setting, and in some areas voluntary agencies offer limited work opportunities and training.

Concrete services might include the provision of equipment, such as canes, walkers, wheelchairs, and hoyer lifts. These may be obtained through the equipment loan programs of the local MS Society chapters. Some churches and fraternal organizations such as the Rotary, Elks, and Kiwanis may also have equipment available.

Homemaker and housekeeping services, transportation, and modifications to make a home accessible and barrier-free may be available through local community agencies and volunteer programs. Information about specialized services, such as hand controls and dwelling modifications, is available through rehabilitation centers and departments of physical and rehabilitation medicine in medical centers.

Talking books constitute another resource now more readily available to MS persons who have blurred or double vision, suffer from extreme weakness or excessive fatigue, are unable to hold a book or turn pages, or have other physical limitations that render them unable to read standard printed books. The limiting condition must be certified by a professional such as a physician, social worker, rehabilitation counselor, nurse, or therapist. Local public libraries and local chapters of the MS Society as well as the Division for the Blind and Physically Handicapped in the Library of Congress can supply more detailed information and application forms.

Education about MS—its symptoms, management, and the physical and emotional problems of daily living—is of considerable importance and should not be neglected in a chapter on care for the MS patient and family. Informal education must be considered a major resource. This involves actively soliciting information during medical visits, particularly where MS care is provided by a team with multiple professional disciplines represented. Literature about MS, problems of living with the illness, and some available services and resources are available through the National Multiple Sclerosis Society and its chapters. More formal educational programs are being developed by local MS chapters themselves and in conjunction with professional organizations, such as medical societies and nursing associations. The MS Homecare Course, developed in conjunction with the American Red Cross, continues to be taught by MS chapters throughout the country. This is oriented primarily to the MS family and deals with many areas of patient care.

It is important to note that all of the resources discussed in this section, even some of the governmental programs, vary considerably from area to area. Eligibility for programs and services is a major consideration, being based on financial as well as physical factors, and must be investigated on an individual case basis. Where questions exist as to the availability of services in a given area, there are some basic sources of information that can be helpful. These include the local MS Society chapters who maintain a community resource file as part of their basic programs, Community Councils, community resource directories, hospital social service departments, and professional associations such as the local medical societies.

A chapter in a book such as this one seeks to apply theoretical formulations to the realities of seeking and providing care. With the knowledge base presented, one should be better prepared to obtain available resources in one's localities.

APPENDIX A: SOCIAL SECURITY ADMINISTRATION PAMPHLETS FOR THE DISABLED

A Brief Explanation of Medicare, HCFA, SSA Publication No. 05-10043.

A Guide to Supplemental Security Income, SSA, SSA Publication No. 05-11015.

A Message From Social Security: Why a Special Medical Examination Is Needed for Your Disability Claim. HHS Publication No. (SSA) 05-10087.

A Woman's Guide to Social Security. HHS Publication No. (SSA) 05-10127.

If You Become Disabled. HHS Publication No. (SSA) 05-10029.

Right to Appeal Supplemental Security Income. HHS Publication No. (SSA) 05-10281.

Right to Appeal Under Social Security and Medicare. HHS Publication No. (SSA) 05-10282.

Social Security Credits—How You Earn Them. SSA, SSA Publication No. 05-10072.

Vocational Rehabilitation for the Blind and Disabled. HHS Publication No. (SSA) 05-10094.

Your Medicare Handbook. HHS Publication No. (SSA) 05-10050.

Your Social Security. HHS Publication No. (SSA) 05-10035.

Your Social Security Rights and Responsibilities: Disability Benefits. HHS Publication No. (SSA) 05-10153.

SSI for Aged, Disabled, and Blind People. HHS Publication No. 05-11000.

Annotated Bibliography

1. MS (1977): *Brit. Med. Bull.*, 33:1.

This was a "state of the art" volume of this journal as of the beginning of 1977. While much of the material on lymphocytes and immunology of MS, and treatment are dated, the chapters on pathology of the MS lesion, and diagnosis and epidemiology of MS, remain useful.

2. Hallpike, J. F., Adams, C. W. M., and Tourtellotte, W. W. (editors) (1983): *Multiple Sclerosis*. Chapman & Hall, London.

This is the latest, most comprehensive volume on MS written for the health professional. Basic science topics include basic pathophysiology and biochemistry of myelin and the demyelinating process, and the most recent immunologic knowledge about MS. Clinical subjects include diagnostic modalities, clinical manifestations and epidemiology, and treatment rationale. The book is heavily referenced and is an excellent reference source.

3. Antel, J. P., and Aranson, B. G. (1980): MS and Other Demyelinating Disease. In *Harrison Principles of Internal Medicine*, 9th ed. McGraw Hill, New York.

This is a good introductory chapter to MS for the non-neurologist. It briefly covers the pathology, epidemiology, and clinical manifestations of the disease. The sections on immunology and laboratory tests are not as current as they could be and therefore are somewhat incomplete. The best sections are those on clinical manifestations and differential diagnosis. The references at the end of the chapter are limited.

4. Wyngarden, J. B., and Smith, L. M. (editors) (1982): The Demyelinating Diseases. In *Cecil—Textbook of Medicine*, 16th ed. W. B. Saunders, Philadelphia.

This brief chapter will serve as a somewhat superficial introduction to multiple sclerosis. The section on therapeutics is well done, although the space allotted to clinical manifestations of the disease is too brief. Nothing is said about the immunopathology of the disease. The references at the end of the chapter are varied and current and include recent immunological advances.

5. Adams, R. O., and Victor, M. (1981): Multiple Sclerosis and Allied Demyelinative Diseases. In *Principles of Neurology*, 2nd ed. McGraw Hill, New York.

This is an excellent and detailed description of MS. The epidemiologic and clinical sections are particularly informative, and include some of the less common variants of the disease. The references at the end of the chapter are extensive and cover a wide range of immunologic, epidemiologic, and clinical material.

6. McFarlin, D. E., and McFarland, H. F. (1982): Multiple Sclerosis. *New Engl. J. Med.*, 307:1183 and 307:1246.

These two articles are an excellent summary of the current epidemiologic and basic science literature on MS. Part I details the most recent immunopathologic findings in MS and their possible clinical applications. Part II describes some of the virologic and epidemiologic knowledge to date and discusses some of the hypotheses about the etiology of MS that have arisen from them. There are a large number of references for each article.

7. Multiple Sclerosis Update (1980): *Neurology*, 30 (7):1–123.

This symposium devoted to MS covers the clinical, therapeutic, basic science, and long-term care aspects of the disease. The sections on management of bladder problems and spasticity are particularly well done, as are the articles on the viral theories of etiology of MS. There is also an excellent chapter on the use of evoked potentials for diagnosis.

Subject Index